THE
WOMEN'S
MIGRAINE
SURVIVAL GUIDE

THE
WOMEN'S
MIGRAINE
SURVIVAL GUIDE

The most complete, up-to-date resource on the causes of your migraine pain—and treatments for real relief

CHRISTINA PETERSON, M.D.

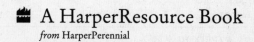
A HarperResource Book
from HarperPerennial

HarperCollins books may be purchased for educational, business, or sales promotional use. For information please write: Special Markets Department, HarperCollins Publishers, Inc., 10 East 53rd Street, New York, NY 10022.

FIRST EDITION

Designed by Stanley S. Drate/Folio Graphics Co. Inc.

Library of Congress Cataloging-in-Publication Data
Peterson, Christina.
    The women's migraine survival guide: the most complete, up-to-
    date resource on the causes of your migraine pain—and treatments
    for real relief / Christina Peterson.
        p.   cm.
    Includes index.
    ISBN 0-06-095319-5
    1. Migraine Popular works.   2. Women—Diseases Popular works.
I. Title.
RC392.P445   1999
616.8'57'0082—dc21   99-27288

99 00 01 02 03 ❖/RRD 10 9 8 7 6 5 4 3 2 1

Contents

Acknowledgments

I would like to especially thank Wanda Urbanska for her extensive assistance with the manuscript. Thanks also go to Chris Adamec for her assistance with the initial concept and proposal for this book. I would like to thank Susan Weinberg, publishing director, and Jen Hart, director of marketing at HarperPerennial for supporting this project. Thanks also to Mike Bradley for technical advice on this project. Sincere thanks go to Peggy Tucker for cheerfully putting up with the endless faxes and other intrusions into the office caused by "The Book." Thanks to all the friends and family who supported this endeavor, and tolerated the vast amounts of time it consumed. Thanks to all the patients who enthusiastically urged me on, and from whom I continue to learn about migraine. And most especially, thanks to Laureen Rowland, my editor, for superb guidance of a first-time author through the labyrinths of the publishing world.

THE
WOMEN'S
MIGRAINE
SURVIVAL GUIDE

———————◆×◆———————

What Is Migraine?

Her migraine came on without much warning, leaving Amy temporarily paralyzed. It felt like a vise tightening around her head, delivering a steady, throbbing pain interrupted only by the jackhammer drilling into one side of her skull. Amy couldn't go to work; she couldn't even leave the bedroom. In fact, the only thing she could do was to lay perfectly still on her bed in the dark; the slightest movement or trace of light or sound would deepen and intensify the pain.

This headache was worse than the one before it, but Amy was no stranger to the pain of migraine. She'd been down this excruciating road many times before. As she lay there feeling comatose, Amy thought back to the first migraine she'd had as a young child. It hurt so badly that she'd begged her mom to chop off her head. If her mother were here today, she'd probably ask for the same mercy—anything to put her out of her misery.

If you're a woman who suffers from migraines, it's likely your experience resembles Amy's. It may provide you with some small measure of comfort to know that you're not alone—in fact, millions share your pain. And while men do get migraine, this is no equal-opportunity disease. Of the estimated 23 million migraine sufferers or "migraineurs" in this country, 18 million are female. Most experts cite a lifetime ratio of three to one for female to male migraineurs.

Just which women are most prone to migraine?

They are women just like—and including—you and me. Though migraine can afflict people in just about any age group, from toddlers through the elderly, its most typical victim is a woman in her childbearing years, with one study showing women in their forties to have the highest incidence. And while people from every racial group are prone to "brain pain" (as migraine is often called), Caucasian women are somewhat more likely than African-American and Asian-American women to suffer. Recent studies show that those living in rural areas are slightly more likely to suffer from migraine than those living in major metropolitan areas. And it's long been established that migraine tends to run in families. If your mother, grandmother, or uncle had them, you're more likely to get migraine than someone with no family history of the illness. Although no one is sure why this is true, recent studies—contradicting earlier ones—show migraine to be more prevalent among individuals with less formal education than among those with college degrees. Despite all these likelihoods, however, we know that migraine afflicts individuals of all ages, racial groups, economic segments, and professions.

Although I am a neurologist specializing in migraine and headache care who's knowledgeable about the most advanced medical and pharmaceutical developments and breakthroughs in migraine research, even I am not immune to the strickening power of these vicious, throbbing headaches. In fact, I have suffered from the anguish of migraines since I was twelve years old. So prominently have they figured in my life that when I sat down to take my neurology boards, I was hit by a migraine. Sick to my stomach, my head pounding, I had no choice but to leave the room.

In this chapter I'll provide an overview of migraine and its key symptoms, lay out the different kinds of migraines, cover some theories on its causes, and review twelve common myths and facts associated with migraine. You can complete a questionnaire to help you determine whether what you're having is really a migraine or if it's another kind of monkey. In addition, I will discuss why women are more prone to migraine than men and touch on—get ready for this—the "good" news about migraine.

If you find that you do suffer from migraine, let me reassure you, both from the perspective of a physician and that of a fellow migraineur, there *are* ways of preventing these headaches and of treating the pain when a migraine does strike. I'll share insights with you about how I manage my own migraines. My goal in this book is to help you to cope effectively with yours.

In later chapters I'll discuss the quantum improvements provided by new medications prescribed for migraine, many of which have just been introduced. They work for many women, including some who have found little or no pain relief from previous medications. Some of these new medications have the advantage of working very quickly—often in a matter of minutes—enabling women to maintain a normal life and not have to "stand down" and lose precious hours and days every time a migraine hits.

I'll also provide the latest information on alternative treatments for pain relief—from massage and acupuncture to aromatherapy and herbal remedies. Some of these solutions may never have occurred to you before and may greatly reduce both your pain and your incidences of migraine.

Perhaps even more significant, I will arm you with as much knowledge as possible to prepare yourself for the onset of a debilitating migraine. You may even be surprised to discover that preventive strategies described in this book—ranging from keeping a migraine diary to recognizing and avoiding your personal food, hormonal, and lifestyle migraine triggers—will provide you with the best arsenal of relief yet.

BUT IT'S "JUST A HEADACHE"!

No doubt you've heard this aggravating phrase countless times before—perhaps from your friends, your boss, your coworkers, maybe even your spouse and children. To those people who think "it's just a headache," the obvious solution for you is to simply pop two aspirins (or some other over-the-counter painkiller) and get on with your life. Clearly, these people have never experienced the debilitating pain of migraine; they just don't get it.

"People hear the word *headache* and immediately think 'Tylenol,' " said Cindy, thirty-one, a patient and migraine sufferer for almost twenty years. "And I think, oh, terrific! A Band-Aid for a bullet wound!"

As one who experiences them all too well knows, migraines are rarely so easily dispatched. Here's how Lucy, age twenty-eight, put it: "A migraine is like a freight train, a rugby game, and a mining operation, all going on and through your head at once."

Unlike the minor and temporary headaches that others are thinking of when they urge you to take a few aspirins, migraine not only is more severe but has a far greater impact. As hard as you might fight them, experiencing multiple migraines over time robs you of hours and days from your work and family life. It's not uncommon to find yourself canceling an eagerly awaited vacation or dinner party because you are physically incapable of going. You relinquish control of your life.

Many women with migraines feel sad and resentful about losing large chunks of their lives. "One of the hardest things about migraines for me is having my life put on hold while I wait for the headache to be over," said Carol, thirty-four, a patient who has suffered from migraine since age fifteen.

Laura, twenty-nine, who has suffered from migraines since age twelve, adds, "One of the worst parts is the fear of *when* it will rear its ugly head. You never know when you're going to lose twenty-four or forty-eight hours. Where am I going to be when it hits? Will I be driving a car? At my sister's wedding? It's the not knowing that's almost worse than the pain."

Women I've spoken with, both in my practice and at the speaking engagements that I regularly give throughout the country, also describe the "waiting-for-the-other-shoe-to-drop" feeling, causing them to virtually center their lives around possible signs of an oncoming attack. In fact, studies of women with migraines reveal that nearly one-third report that their lives are dominated by the dread of their next migraine.

Migraines cannot and should not define our lives. I've written this book to help put the migraine in its place—and to return you to where you belong, at the helm and in control of your life, doing the things you need and love to do and doing them when *you* want to, not at the whim of your migraines.

IS THIS YOU?

How do you know if you suffer from migraines? Check the following scenario against your own experience with headaches.

You're ready to head off for what you hope will be an idyllic family vacation. You've been looking forward to this trip for what seems like forever. You've made plans, confirmed your reservations, given the dog sitter instructions, and just put away that last report. At last, the promised land is in sight!

But then you start to notice the lights in the living room are bothering you—did they suddenly become brighter? Maybe someone put in a new, higher-wattage lightbulb. But there's a halo around the halogen lamp too, which wasn't there last night.

Maybe you're just tired. Or stressed-out. After all, you just worked fifteen extra hours over three days in order to be able to enjoy this trip. It's certainly about time that you enjoyed some well-deserved R&R. And yet, the more you try to deny that your head is starting to feel strange, the more you notice that nauseated sensation bubbling up in your stomach. Yes, it's a migraine. And in almost no time you're lying statue-still, flat on your back, in your room, lights off, shades drawn. You beg your family to go without you. You'll meet up with them later when you're better. But they won't budge. Mom's sick; the trip is off. "How come you always get a headache when we've got something fun planned?" your children ask you.

Guilt and anguish compound the piercing, all-consuming pain.

Or take thirty-one-year-old Ashley. Her period is due in a few days, and like clockwork, her head begins pounding. She feels nauseated. Her neck hurts. She can't sit up. She can't drive to work. And she doesn't understand why this has to happen to her every single month.

AN UNRECOGNIZED AFFLICTION

If you're reading this book, you either know or suspect that you or someone you care about has migraines. The fact is, many women suffer in silence, undiagnosed and untreated.

A recent study conducted by Innovative Medical Research and led by noted headache researcher Richard Lipton, M.D., a neurologist at the Albert Einstein College of Medicine in New York City, showed that of the 31,000 people interviewed, nearly 3,100, or about 10 percent, had headaches that could be classified as migraines, according to the International Headache Society. Yet nearly half of this 10 percent had no idea that what they were experiencing was migraine!

These unwitting migraineurs had "diagnosed" themselves with "sinus headaches" or "stress headaches." The symptoms they reported, as well as their descriptions of the pain, clearly revealed that their problem was really migraines. "Excruciatingly intense," "headbanger," and "hellish" were some of the terms they used. Perhaps even more significant, the researchers discovered that younger people (under age thirty) were less likely to identify their headaches as migraines and more likely to simply shrug them off as "stress," whereas many people over thirty wrongly believed they were suffering from sinus problems. Not surprisingly, most of the women surveyed were also quick to link their headaches with stress.

But in many significant ways, a migraine is very different from other kinds of headaches, including stress and sinus headaches. Here's how to know if you're suffering from migraine.

IS IT MIGRAINE? TEST YOURSELF

Here are a few questions for you to consider in determining whether your headaches are migraines. (To be sure it's migraine, have a physician evaluate you.) Answer true or false to the following questions:

	T	F
1. My headaches are severe and pounding.	☐	☐
2. I often feel nauseous during a headache attack.	☐	☐
3. The headaches come before or during my period.	☐	☐
4. My mother or my sister (or daughter or father) has the same kind of headaches.	☐	☐
5. I have missed work or important events because of my headaches.	☐	☐

	T	F
6. I can't stand any light or noise when I have a bad headache.	☐	☐
7. Moving around too much or bending over can make the pain worse.	☐	☐
8. The pain is often on one side of my head.	☐	☐
9. Tylenol or aspirin doesn't help much (or not at all).	☐	☐
10. My headache can last from about five hours to several days.	☐	☐

If you answered "true" to more than three of these questions, you may indeed be suffering from migraines. If you answered "true" to six or more, then you probably do have migraines. Have your doctor make the final analysis.

If you think you may be experiencing migraines, it will help a lot to understand precisely what a migraine is. You know it's an intense headache. But what else is involved?

MAJOR KINDS OF MIGRAINE

Migraines are divided into two broad categories: those that are preceded by a warning, or an "aura," and those that are not. In the past the former type has been called the "classic migraine" and the latter, the "common migraine." Whether or not the migraine comes with a warning, you'll know when the head pain hits—it'll feel like a freight train charging through your brain.

LIGHT SHOW

About 15 to 20 percent of migraine sufferers experience an aura, which is a neurologic symptom that usually affects vision on one side of the body and precedes the head pain. As a result, some women who experience auras have a window of time before the head pain starts in which to take medication. An aura may last up to an hour, but most range from five to thirty minutes and can continue as the head pain occurs. Many women who experience auras find that they involve some sort of visual change. Some migraineurs see flashing lights or lightning bolts, often at the edge of their visual field.

Others develop what is called a scotoma—a blank spot of missing vision that often occurs in the center of the visual field. Tunnel vision can also occur. Complex visual phenomena have also been described in migraine auras, often involving linear aspects, such as a "picket fence" pattern or zigzags. Colored spots or shapes may appear. Crescent shapes— especially at the edges of vision—are often reported.

Some migraineurs experience blurred vision. Rarely, very complex and even surrealistic apparitions may occur. One migraineur I know reported seeing either the painting *Blue Boy* or four red roses from a whiskey ad as her migraine aura!

Auras can also involve nonvisual symptoms. The most common of these is paresthesia, which is a numbness or tingling feeling, usually felt in the arm or face or both. "I get a pins-and-needles kind of prickly feeling in my face before the migraine pain hits me," says Lana, thirty-five.

Weakness or slurring of speech can also occur as part of the aura, although this symptom is less frequent than paresthesia. Weakness or numbness in the arm may occur; the same symptoms can occur in the leg, but much less commonly. Rarely, an aura can render a person unable to formulate words or sentences; this strokelike symptom can be very alarming.

After the aura phase, the pain begins. Head pain can occur either on the same side as the aura or on the opposite side. While many migraines are unilateral, some occur on both sides of the head. The most common pain sites are the areas around and behind the eyes, the temples, or the back of the head. Pain may even move around the head during an attack.

Throughout the course of the headache, loud sounds, bright lights, or strong odors may be intolerable. The pain is often made worse by even simple exertion, such as walking up a flight of stairs.

MIGRAINE WITHOUT AURA

Migraine without aura is like migraine with aura, except there is no symptomatic warning phase. There may be a vague period of warning, however. This is called a prodrome, and it can occur hours before a migraine, or even on the preceding day. The prodrome can include the following symptoms:

- food cravings
- lack of appetite
- increased thirst
- fluid retention
- increased urination
- constipation or diarrhea
- yawning
- difficulty concentrating
- restlessness
- drowsiness
- depression
- coldness

Given a list like that, you might think you have a migraine coming on *every* day. But once you're aware of these symptoms and how they manifest themselves in you, then you can learn to differentiate them—for example, distinguishing "normal" hunger from your premigraine hunger.

"I'll become very tired or hungry before a migraine. Sometimes my nose becomes congested on the side that the headache is about to start on," said Jerri, thirty-four, a migraine patient of mine for many years.

"I have several hints that a migraine is coming," said Jane, forty-five, a long-term migraineur. "Excessive urination and excessive yawning are two of them. I also seem to have either a lot more or a lot less energy than usual. Sometimes I am in a black mood beforehand."

Claudia, twenty-nine, says she feels "out of it" before a migraine. "For me, there's a feeling of unreality about things, a bit like when you first wake up in the morning and you're not quite awake yet."

Eva, forty-one, has noted a pattern before her migraines hit. "Usually I start feeling warm, very dry, and very thirsty. Sometimes I notice myself feeling kind of irrationally hostile shortly before a bad migraine comes."

Prodromes can last minutes to hours and thus don't offer a reliable indication of when to take medication. In Chapter 2 we'll discuss the importance of noting prodromes in your migraine diary as a way of preparing for and preventing migraines.

WHAT DOES A MIGRAINE FEEL LIKE?

Of course, migraines vary from individual to individual, but there are characteristic migraine symptoms that can tip you off to the onset. These include:

- head pain
- nausea
- vomiting
- sensitivity to light
- sensitivity to sound
- sensitivity to odors and touch
- dizziness
- inability to concentrate

HEAD PAIN AND NAUSEA

Most migraineurs experience severe head pain during a migraine attack, and this is usually the worst symptom. It can be blinding and is often described as throbbing, or occurring in waves. It often affects half the head, or it can be centered in one spot like a glowing ember. Occasionally, migraine pain will involve the entire head.

Nausea—sometimes accompanied by vomiting—is another common element of migraine. It's also a problem for many women who don't have sufficient warning that a migraine is coming on and can't take medication before the nausea begins. Once the nausea hits, digestion ceases or slows to the point that any pills taken will not be absorbed for hours, even if you do not vomit. (For this reason, migraine medications come in several forms other than pills. That information is covered in Chapter 7.)

VOMITING

If you are vomiting repeatedly, you may become dehydrated. You may also be losing electrolytes and should try to drink plenty of fluids. Should vomiting persist for more than eighteen hours, call your doctor for guidance.

After the migraine has passed, you may find yourself extremely thirsty. One patient said that she drinks large quantities of Gatorade after a migraine. Normally she can't stand the taste of the stuff, but after a migraine, it tastes like nectar. Pedialyte, available in the infant-care sections of most pharmacies, can also help replace electrolytes.

SENSITIVITY TO LIGHT AND SOUND

Many women with migraines report that even normal levels of light bother them during an attack. And some migraineurs find even standard levels of sound extremely irritating as well. Photophobia (sensitivity to light) and phonophobia, also known as sonophobia (sensitivity to sound), have been documented in many clinical studies of migraineurs. We'll discuss these symptoms in depth later in the book; the best ways to address such sensitivities are also the most obvious: wear sunglasses outside; draw the draperies or blinds in your home; keep the television or stereo volume low; wear earplugs.

SENSITIVITY TO ODOR AND TOUCH

You may be among the women who, when experiencing a migraine, are hypersensitive to odors. Dolores, thirty-seven, confided that her husband and son eat all their meals out whenever she has a migraine, so that kitchen odors won't aggravate her pain. For their considerate behavior, she says, they have earned a "migraine medal" in her book. Jill, forty-eight, who has experienced migraines since puberty, said, "When you have the headache, even paper has a smell. And smells can be so intense as to be devastating."

Others find that during a migraine they are hypersensitive to touch. Even the lightest touch, which would otherwise be a welcome caress, may be positively painful while in the throes of a migraine. One woman who has suffered from migraines for years joked that it's always "best to let sleeping migraineurs lie."

DIZZINESS AND INABILITY TO CONCENTRATE

Some women report a feeling of vertigo or motion sickness with migraine. Along with the dizziness, many women have difficulty concentrating through a migraine. In fact, some migraineurs have said that the overall confusion or inability to concentrate is nearly as debilitating as the pain itself.

WHAT CAUSES A MIGRAINE?

As a physician, I am naturally analytical, seeking the root cause in order to explain the effect. That's why migraine treatment can be so frustrating. The fact is, the medical profession really doesn't know exactly how or why migraines begin. However, we do have some clues. Recent research has indicated that migraines are "born" in the area of the brain known as the brainstem; as the migraine develops, alterations in the brain's physiology ensue.

For example, blood flow to the brain decreases slightly. This decrease begins at the back of the brain and spreads forward at about two to three millimeters per minute. After this process begins, women who experience auras will enter their aura phase. Whether or not you are an "aura person," this decreased blood flow is followed by the beginning of the headache phase. While the headache is still going strong, blood flow to the brain tissue increases slightly. The increase in blood flow persists for a while after the headache subsides. Experts don't think that these minor alterations cause either the aura or the pain of a migraine. Instead, most now believe it is the abnormal functioning of brain cells, not a lack of blood supply, that causes the migraine aura.

The blood vessels on the brain's surface (meningeal vessels) expand when you have a migraine, and this dilation is likely to be the cause of the pain. A fine network of nerves supplies these blood vessels. When the vessels dilate, these nerves are then tipped off and instructed to throb with pain.

At a biochemical level, scientists know that several neurotransmitters are released during a migraine. Experts in migraine also know that medications that influence serotonin receptors—thereby increasing the level of serotonin in the brain—can help reverse this blood-vessel dilation and subsequently relieve migraine pain, nausea, and the other symptoms.

It would seem logical, then, for all migraine sufferers to simply alter the level of serotonin in their brain, either through medication or diet. But it isn't that simple. Why not? Because your brain is very carefully protected from your bloodstream, in order to keep it safe from toxins.

There are two primary ways that medications, vitamins, or hormones can reach the brain. They must either travel through special channels in the blood-vessel wall or be brought in by a special "carrier" protein. The special channels have biochemical "gates" that act as filters to control what gets through. This means that taking an oral form of a neurotransmitter will generally not help, unless the body has a mechanism to usher it through the blood/brain barrier and into the brain.

Thus, taking a serotonin precursor (available at many health food stores under the names of tryptamine, hydroxy-tryptamine, or 5HTP) won't help, either as a preventative to migraine or as a painkiller. But there are medications that can penetrate the filter and boost your serotonin level; these can be prescribed by your physician.

COULD IT BE BACTERIAL?

One Italian study has indicated that *Helicobacter pylori*, the same bacteria that causes most stomach ulcers, could also be implicated in migraines. In 1998 Dr. A. Gasbarrini and his colleagues at Catholic University in Rome reported on their attempt to link *H. pylori* to migraines. They found that 40 percent of their 225 patients with migraine also tested positive for *H. pylori*. The infected patients were then treated with appropriate antibiotics, and in the majority of cases, the *H. pylori* was eradicated. The exciting news: Elimination of the *H. pylori* was followed by a significant reduction in the frequency and severity of the subjects' migraines.

While it is unlikely that *Helicobacter pylori* was the cause of the migraines, it may have served as a trigger, lowering the migraineurs' physiological threshold and predisposing them to a greater occurrence of migraine attacks. If that is the case, then removing the offending agent (in this case, *H. pylori)* would result in fewer migraines.

Of course, one study alone is not enough from which to draw broad-based conclusions, and you should not rush out to insist that your doctor test you for *H. pylori*. However, physicians and researchers specializing in migraine science are pursuing this link and probing for further information.

MAGNESIUM DEFICIENCY?

Some studies have noted that migraineurs show lower levels of magnesium during a migraine. However, low magnesium in general has not been conclusively linked to migraine, although researchers suspect there may be a subset of migraineurs who experience low magnesium levels even between migraines. So migraine isn't simply the result of a magnesium deficiency. Rather, it is more likely that reduced magnesium within the cells makes nerve-cell membranes unstable, leaving the brain susceptible to developing a migraine.

WHY WOMEN MORE THAN MEN?

Migraines are more prevalent among women than men for three reasons: hormonal changes, genetic susceptibility, and increased levels of stress. Let's examine these reasons in more detail.

WHAT'S FEMALE BIOLOGY GOT TO DO WITH IT?

If you're still menstruating, monthly hormonal shifts could be triggering your migraine headaches. A clue that hormonal shifts may be a factor is if your headaches occur just before your period or during menstruation; this is the case for 60 percent of women with migraines.

Other events causing female hormonal shifts, such as pregnancy or menopause, can directly affect your migraines, causing them to decrease, subside, or become more frequent. Of course, there are also variations from woman to woman, even at the same ages and stages. For example, during pregnancy, some women experience a decrease in migraines; others experience migraine for the first time.

Sometimes hormones that we introduce into our bodies can affect our probability for migraine. For example, oral contraceptives (all of which contain hormones) can trigger migraines in some women, while others are unaffected. Hormone replacement therapy (HRT) may alleviate migraines in some menopausal women, exacerbate them in others. Menstruation, pregnancy, and menopausal migraines are major complaints among women with migraines. I devote a full chapter to each subject later in the book.

BLAME IT ON YOUR GENES

Studies comparing twins raised together with twins raised apart have been performed for years in many countries and have clearly established that migraine runs in families. Even without twin studies, we know genetics is important: For example, research has revealed that if both your parents experienced migraines, your probability of getting migraines is about 70 percent. If your parents didn't suffer from migraines and you do, a careful survey of aunts, uncles, cousins, and grandparents will probably yield a history of "sick headaches," or migraine.

But why is it that females, so much more than males, are saddled with migraine headaches? Though there is no conclusive evidence, the cause may be related to estrogen. Prior to puberty, boys and girls experience migraines in equal numbers. After puberty, migraine is a far greater problem for women, and that three-to-one ratio kicks in.

Another link to genetic causation involves a rare form of migraine known as familial hemiplegic migraine. Scientists have found that the gene that causes this migraine may "live" on either chromosome 19 or chromosome 1. Does it stand to reason, then, that the gene for "regular" migraines could "live" on either one of these chromosomes—or perhaps another? It's possible. Or the genetic causes may be found in another place altogether or perhaps in several places. Research is proceeding at a rapid rate; only time will tell.

THE SUPERWOMAN SYNDROME

If you're raising a family, maintaining a household, *and* holding down a full-time job, that doesn't leave a lot of time to be down with a migraine. Torn between work demands ("The project is due today"), family demands ("Your son is sick; come pick him up at school"), marital demands ("Listen to my problems"), and elderly demands ("I'm afraid you're going to put me in a nursing home"), it's no wonder many women today find themselves feeling stress overload.

If you don't have a propensity for getting migraines, such stresses are unlikely to cause them. However, if you do have that tendency, then stress can be trigger number one for you.

COULD IT BE ANOTHER KIND OF HEADACHE?

Sometimes the problem is *not* migraine, even though your head hurts something awful and you may have other symptoms that suggest migraine. There are more than three hundred causes of headaches; some of the best known, as well as several rare but interesting headaches, are covered here.

TENSION-TYPE HEADACHES

You have probably heard the term "tension headache," which refers to the most common headache there is. Some doctors refer to it as "muscle-contraction headache." Most people—even those who don't experience headaches regularly—have had a tension-type headache at some point in their lives.

Is this a headache that occurs when you're stressed-out? Sometimes, but that's not what the term means. In fact, doctors changed the name of this headache category from "tension headache" to "tension-type headache" to get away from the idea that stress or psychological problems are the sole causes.

Tension-type headaches can be brought on by stress or tension as well as lack of sleep (as can migraine). These headaches may also result from neck problems or poor posture. Sometimes jaw or dental problems can induce tension-type headaches as well as oral and facial pain.

The bad news for women: According to a Johns Hopkins study reported in 1998, women experience 15 percent more tension-type headaches than men do. It might be a hormonal issue, because many report that the headaches occur around menstruation. But there's no clearly demonstrated association between this kind of headache and menstruation.

Tension-type headaches are most common among thirty- to thirty-nine-year-olds. This doesn't mean that if you're forty-five, you can't get a tension-type headache. You can. It's just less likely. As with migraine, the prevalence of tension-type headaches decreases with age.

How does a tension-type headache differ from a migraine? First, the pain of tension-type headache is usually not one-sided. It's a pressure, squeezing, or tight kind of pain, whereas migraine pain is usually pulsating or throbbing. Tension-type headaches, which are of mild to moderate intensity, are not worsened by exertion such as climbing stairs. Nor are they associated with nausea or vomiting. The person suffering from a tension-type headache doesn't usually avoid bright lights or loud sounds.

Migraine sufferers can also experience tension-type headaches. In fact, some headache specialists consider tension-type headache and migraine to be different facets of the same thing, probably due to the same biochemical brain abnormalities.

Very few tension-type headache sufferers—less than 20 percent—have seen a physician about their headaches. This is unfortunate, because there are medications and treatments that can help. If you or someone you know has chronic tension-type headaches, I urge you or your friend to seek medical attention.

In case you're still uncertain as to which headache is which, the following chart will help you differentiate between migraine and tension-type headaches:

TENSION-TYPE VS. MIGRAINE

	Tension-type headache	Migraine
One-sided pain?	No	Usually
Pressure pain?	Yes	No
Throbbing pain?	No	Yes
Exertion worsens headache?	No	Yes
Intensity?	Mild to moderate	Moderate to severe
Nausea and/or vomiting?	No	Yes
Need to avoid bright lights?	No	Yes
Need to avoid loud noises?	No	Yes
Headache responds to acetaminophen or ibuprofen?	Yes, generally	Not usually

MIXED HEADACHE

Sometimes your headache has the features of one category, such as migraine, along with features of another headache category, such as tension-type. For example, Alicia, forty-one, has headaches that involve more pressure pain than throbbing, which would make her doctor lean toward diagnosing a tension-type headache. But loud sounds bother her terribly during a headache—a migraine indicator. Further complicating the diagnosis, Alicia is never nauseated during a headache, as many migraineurs are. And mild exercise doesn't make the headache any worse—tension-type. On the other hand, her pain is quite severe. "I can't think straight during one of these!" she asserted. Back to migraine.

Alicia suffers from what's called the mixed headache. The terms "tension-vascular headache," "combined headache," and "combination headache" have also been used to denote the headache with features of both migraine and tension-type. It doesn't quite fit the criteria for a migraine headache, but it's too much like a migraine to be classified as tension-type headache.

Some experts would tell Alicia that migraine and tension-type headaches actually exhibit more similarities than differences, and they'd talk to her about a continuum theory of headache. The mixed headache would fall in the center of the spectrum.

If they're right about a headache continuum, this may explain why studies have shown that Imitrex, one of the revolutionary new antimigraine medications, relieves tension-type headaches in migraine sufferers. (Imitrex and other triptan medications should never be used to diagnose migraine; just because it works doesn't prove it's a migraine.) On the other hand, tension-type headache does not respond to all the same medications that relieve migraine. Nor does it follow the same genetic inheritance patterns.

REBOUND HEADACHES

Can you develop a headache by taking medicine for your headache? It sounds ridiculous, but unfortunately, it can happen. It's called a rebound headache. It's very painful and often occurs in the morning. People who experience rebound headaches have unknowingly trapped themselves into getting more headaches. How? By taking acetaminophen, aspirin, medications with caffeine, or narcotic painkillers more than three times a week.

The appropriate treatment is obvious: Withdraw the offending medication. But that's not as simple as it sounds. When you stop taking the medication that is both cause and cure of your headaches, the consequence is often severe pain until your body adjusts. When the choice is some pain (caused by the rebound headache and temporarily cured by the offending medication) or very bad pain (caused by not taking the offending medication), many people prefer some pain. Unfortunately, in this case, that is not the best course.

To get off the rebound-headache treadmill, you must stop taking the medication that causes it. Rebound headache can be reversed, through various treatment strategies. If your physician is uncomfortable treating the rebound headache—which is, after all, a highly specialized problem—a neurologist or physician at a headache clinic is equipped to handle it.

The best strategy is to avoid the problem in the first place. Take medication, including over-the-counter drugs, only as directed by your physician.

HEAD INJURY

If you are unfortunate enough to have experienced a head injury, especially one with a concussion, you may have headaches for a period of time after the injury. Sometimes this posttraumatic headache has features of a migraine. If you already had migraines before the head injury, they may worsen as a result of the injury.

With a mild head injury, where there is no prolonged loss of consciousness and no significant brain damage, 80 percent of the headaches that occur will go away within six months.

FEBRILE (FEVER) HEADACHES AND METABOLIC ABNORMALITIES

An infection with fever often causes a headache. Various alterations in the body's metabolism during a fever can bring it on. Studies show that 68 to 100 percent of viral influenza patients experience headaches.

There are also headaches that result from metabolic abnormalities. Why do they happen? Some causes are:

- low oxygen levels, either in the atmosphere you breathe or in your blood, due to anemia or lung disease
- carbon monoxide exposure

- hangovers due to the combined effects of dehydration and toxic byproducts of alcohol consumption
- low blood sugar
- low carbon dioxide levels (usually due to hyperventilation)

MEDICATION AND CHEMICALLY INDUCED HEADACHES

Certain medications, environmental toxins, and substance abuse can induce headaches. Some medications that can cause migraines are Bactrim, Zantac, Prozac, digitalis, and nitroglycerine.

A rarely seen side effect of medication that is prescribed for an acute headache attack—such as sumatriptan (Imitrex) or ergotamine—is actual worsening of headache pain.

"Street" drugs can lead to headaches, and headaches have been reported with the use of cocaine, amphetamine, and marijuana.

Even the inhalation of trace amounts of common household chemicals can lead to a headache in a susceptible migraineur. Exposure to the chemicals carbon disulfide, carbon tetrachloride, camphor, hydrogen sulfide, kerosene, methyl alcohol, naphthalene, nitrous oxide, formaldehyde, and nicotine can trigger headaches. Organophosphate pesticide exposure can also result in headache.

HIGH BLOOD PRESSURE

Very high blood pressure, whether it stems from kidney disease, essential hypertension, or toxemia (preeclampsia) in pregnancy, can cause a headache. Interestingly, high blood pressure is nearly twice as likely to occur in migraineurs as in those unaffected.

If you have high blood pressure, be sure to get some recommendations from your doctor to help you move your blood pressure within the normal range and keep it there.

UNUSUAL HEADACHES

Exercise-Induced Headaches

Occasionally, exercising can bring on a severe headache. When this happens you should seek medical evaluation in order to rule out the possibility of it being something else. Benign exertional headaches can sometimes be avoided by warming up slowly. Exercise-induced headaches also often respond to preventive doses of indomethacin (Indocin).

Cough-Induced Headaches

Coughing headaches—usually described as splitting, explosive, and short-lived, followed by a dull headache for several hours—are more prevalent in men and tend to occur more frequently in people over age forty. Sneezing, lifting, crying, singing, laughing, or straining can also bring on this type of headache. I certainly don't recommend that you refrain from singing, laughing, or crying, although you might consider restricting your lifting and straining activities if you have this type of headache.

Sometimes cough-related headaches are a sign of a brain tumor or another brain abnormality, and your doctor may recommend that you get a magnetic resonance imagery (MRI) or computer-aided tomography (CT) scan. If the scan is negative, then there's no reason to worry about benign cough headache.

Sex-Induced Headaches

Contrary to popular opinion, benign sexual headaches are more common in men than in women. They can occur at any age. Just as it sounds, they're precipitated by sexual activity. If you suffer from this kind of headache, it's sporadic and unpredictable, so you won't know if a sexual encounter will lead to one or not.

The benign sexual headache usually begins with dull pain during sexual excitement and becomes most intense at the point of orgasm.

Ice Cream Headaches

Cold-induced headache, also known as ice cream headache, is well known and more common among migraine sufferers. Eating cold foods such as ice cream very fast can bring on a headache. The pain is brief, lasting less than five minutes. It usually occurs in the middle of the forehead but can hit at the usual site of headache in the migraineur. The longer the cold stimulus is applied to the palate and throat, the more likely this headache is to occur. The best solution? Avoid ice cream or very cold foods altogether. Or try my technique—eat them slowly, savoring each bite.

Chronic Paroxysmal Hemicrania Headaches and Cluster Headaches

The chronic paroxysmal hemicrania headache is similar to the cluster headache with a few key differences. Cluster headaches are more common in men than women and are characterized by severe pain in and around the eye; they "cluster" in time, often occurring the same time each day, with attacks lasting anywhere from fifteen minutes to three hours. By contrast, attacks of chronic paroxysmal hemicrania are shorter and occur primarily in women. The most important feature of this headache is that it responds to a specific nonsteroidal anti-inflammatory medication called indomethacin (Indocin). This very rare headache is almost one hundred times less common than the cluster headache.

TWELVE MIGRAINE MYTHS

Because the general public is largely misinformed about this illness, numerous misconceptions about migraine have entered the popular lore. What follows are twelve of the most common myths about women and migraine. Once you're armed with the facts, you can set the record straight when confronted with such troublesome fallacies.

MYTH 1 • *Women get more migraines than men do because women are more emotional and easier to upset.*

FACT • Women experience more migraines than men do as a result of hormonal differences and genetics and their effect on brain biochemicals. The majority of women— however "emotional" they may be—do *not* get migraines.

MYTH 2 • *Many women bring on migraines to avoid something, like sex or work.*

FACT • Migraine is a disorder of altered physiology. While there may be a subset of women (and men) with subconsciously triggered psychosomatic migraines, the vast majority of migraineurs have no psychological reason for their headaches.

MYTH 3 • *Women who suffer from many migraines probably need to see a psychiatrist or psychologist. They must have some inner conflicts that cause those headaches.*

FACT • Some women with migraines also suffer from emotional problems, and addressing inner conflicts in therapy can reduce migraine frequency and severity. (However, it will not "cure" the underlying migraine tendency in the brain.) Some experts believe that the neurochemical changes that cause migraine can also cause mental disorders, such as depression.

If a woman who experiences migraines also has an emotional problem, she may need to consult with a mental-health professional. But most women who suffer from migraines don't need to see a psychiatrist or psychologist; they just need help in averting migraine attacks and managing their pain.

MYTH 4 • *Women get migraines because they eat bad things, like chocolate.*

FACT • Various foods do act as a trigger in about 25 percent of all migraine sufferers, which means that they *don't* precipitate a headache in the majority of migraineurs. Of that 25 percent, not all women react adversely to chocolate. Some women anecdotally report that chocolate actually makes them feel *better*. Why? Because chocolate contains a caffeine-like substance, which can help alleviate pain in some individuals. Other foods that often trigger migraines are red wine, aged cheese, and dishes prepared with MSG. (More about food triggers later in this chapter.)

MYTH 5 · *If a medication works for one woman's migraines, then it should work for most other women, too.*

FACT · Women are not all made from the same mold. A medication or treatment that works for one woman may not work for the next one. There's a tremendous amount of individual variation in responsiveness to given medications.

MYTH 6 · *Women who get migraines are just plain depressed.*

FACT · A disproportionately high number of women with migraine *are* clinically depressed; however, treating their depression does not cure their migraine. Does the recurring pain of migraine make women feel depressed because migraine is inherently depressing? Or is there another cause of both depression and migraine? Research actively continues to work toward determining the underlying factors of this relationship. It is known that depression places one at increased risk of developing migraines and migraine increases the risk of becoming depressed. But it's important to realize that depression is highly treatable.

MYTH 7 · *Women who get migraines usually have PMS (premenstrual syndrome).*

FACT · The approach of a woman's period triggers migraine in many women. But these women do not necessarily also get PMS. For other women, migraines have nothing to do with their menstrual cycle. Some women who do have PMS do not get migraines.

MYTH 8 • *People who get migraines take a lot of time off from work.*

FACT • People with migraines don't appear to take any more time off from work than people with other chronic ailments. In fact, some people with migraines struggle to stay on the job and actually take *less* time off than people with other disorders.

MYTH 9 • *Women who get "weekend headaches" are avoiding their spouses and families.*

FACT • Unfortunately for migraineurs, many women experience migraines on weekends. This could be because of a change from high levels of stress to lower stress levels. It may also be due to changes in daily habits, such as sleeping patterns and decreased caffeine intake. But few (if any) women get migraines because they want to avoid their families.

MYTH 10 • *Only white women get migraines.*

FACT • Women of all races suffer from migraines, though the prevalence is higher among Caucasian women. One study showed a 20.4 percent rate of migraine among Caucasian women, a 16.2 percent prevalence among African-American women, and a 9.2 percent prevalence among Asian-American women.

MYTH 11 • *If a person tried hard enough, she could shake her headache problem.*

FACT • It is simply not possible to "will away" your tendency to migraine. Many migraineurs try hard to find their migraine triggers and to control the illness. Although many women never seek medical treatment, they do take over-the-counter medication in an attempt to lessen these debilitating headaches.

Much can be done to minimize the frequency and severity of migraines. Recent research has yielded new medications and new ideas about migraine. Doctors have made amazing strides in helping people, but we haven't yet learned to cure people of migraines forever.

MYTH 12 · *Women who get migraines are extremely intelligent, high-achieving, nervous people who have a "migraine personality."*

FACT · Though migraine sufferers like the "extremely intelligent" part of this stereotype, unfortunately, no study supports this idea. Many of the women I've treated were very bright; many were also high achievers. Others were of average aptitude and accomplishment.

The American Migraine Study and other research demonstrate that people from all walks of life are plagued by migraines. But women who are high achievers are more likely to have medical resources available to them, are more likely to consult a physician, and are more likely to speak out about their illness than their less privileged "sisters."

While there is an increase in the incidence of certain psychiatric disorders as concomitant conditions with migraine, it is neither fair nor accurate to describe all women with migraine as having personality abnormalities. Nor is the abnormal personality the *cause* of the migraines; one must have a predisposition to migraines.

THE "GOOD" NEWS ABOUT MIGRAINES

I know, you probably can't imagine the word *good* associated in any way with migraines. But truth be told, if you must suffer from migraines, there is no better time than the present.

Women through the ages have suffered from migraine headaches. But either they had no remedies or their "experts" recommended radical solutions such as drilling holes in their skulls (apparently to release "evil spirits") or making them consume nasty or dangerous potions. For example, our ancestors used such migraine "cures" as silver nitrate (which is toxic), *Datura stramonium* (a poisonous plant), aconite, potassium cyanide, and radioactive thorium.

The Egyptian god Horus reputedly prayed for a substitute head until his one-sided headache passed. Other migraine remedies in the past were such "medications" as garlic implanted under the skin in the temple area of the head (a medieval Arabian treatment), treatment with arsenic (about 150 years ago), or exposure to radioactive thorium (about 100 years ago.)

Fortunately, today no one is going to force you to drink mysterious foul-tasting concoctions or submit to the subcutaneous insertion of garlic cloves into your head. The pharmacological and alternative treatments that are available to you today are far less invasive and far more successful than any used before. (You'll read more about alternative and nonpharmaceutical treatments for migraine in Chapter 8.)

While I can't promise you that your migraines will disappear forever, I can and will provide you with the information you need to limit their frequency and severity. Armed with the advice offered in this survival guide, along with the assistance of your own physician, you can step up to a healthier, happier, and less painful life.

Now you have a basic grasp of what migraines are. But how does your doctor determine whether or not your headache problem really is migraine? In the next chapter I'll discuss how physicians diagnose migraines and offer you important advice on how you can help your doctor to help you.

CHAPTER
2

❖

The Right Doctor:
The First Step to Relief

You may believe that these horrendous headaches plaguing you are indeed migraines but you've never seen a doctor to confirm your suspicions. Or you may know for sure that you *do* suffer from migraines but are stoically trying to wait them out without professional help. In either scenario, putting a physician on the case could be your first step to real relief.

Enlisting a doctor who can treat your migraines—whether she is a neurologist specializing in headaches or an internist who has a solid track record of working with migraineurs—can dramatically enhance the quality of your life. In this chapter I'll share my insights on how to find a good doctor, what to expect in an initial appointment, and how to make the most of your limited time with your new physician. I'll give you ideas about how you can help your doctor help you and will cover the kinds of information that a physician needs to diagnose a headache problem. I'll also give you some insight into the diagnostic process and the factors that go into your headache history—that part of your medical history that concentrates on factors that may contribute to your headaches.

Finally, if you already have a doctor but aren't sure you're getting the best care possible for your migraines, I'll guide you in determining whether you should seek a second opinion or find another doctor.

FINDING A DOCTOR

So you've decided to look for someone to help. If your primary-care physician isn't interested in treating your headaches or lacks the expertise to do so, you may wish to seek care from a neurologist or headache specialist. Bear in mind that not all headache specialists are neurologists; some anesthesiologists, rehabilitation specialists, gynecologists, internists, dentists, and oral surgeons also specialize in the treatment of migraines. The National Headache Foundation (800-843-2256; www.headaches.org) and the American Council for Headache Education (800-255-ACHE; www.achenet.org) both keep lists of member physicians specializing in the treatment of headache who are accepting patient referrals. You might also contact your local county medical society, hospital, or health department for a referral. Finally, ask around. Friends, coworkers, pharmacists, and other physicians may be able to steer you to the right person.

HELPING YOUR DOCTOR HELP YOU

THE GREAT COMMUNICATOR

Let's assume you've found the doctor you want to work with. The first—and best—thing you can do to start the relationship out on a good footing is to be a good communicator. Remember, no matter how accomplished and knowledgeable your physician is, she is not clairvoyant and cannot possibly know as much about you as you do. You are your own best advocate, and when you take an active role in your medical care, you invariably obtain better treatment. Without effective communication with your doctor, she may not get a clear and detailed picture of your problem or understand your treatment preferences. (Indeed, in a nationwide survey of two hundred primary-care physicians, the doctors said that about 30 percent of their patients made diagnosis more difficult by failing to communicate their symptoms adequately.)

Communication is crucial not only for the physician to obtain a complete picture of you as an individual and of your headache symptoms but to help *you* understand your diagnosis and what your doctor expects of you in managing it. Yet it's an accepted fact that patients retain only about 40 percent of what a doctor says to them during an appointment.

How can you increase your retention rate? I have three suggestions:

1. *Block out all distractions* so that you focus your complete attention on what's being said.
2. *Take notes.* If something is unclear, or if your physician uses unfamiliar terminology, review this material at the end of the visit. I know I'd rather clarify a point when a patient is right in front of me than have to play telephone tag with her and then search my memory bank for the context of her questions.
3. *Don't be afraid to ask.* Some patients worry about asking questions because they fear the doctor will think they're stupid. Relax. There are no stupid questions. And we don't expect you to be the expert; that's what we're paid for.

YOUR HEADACHE HISTORY

The diagnosis of migraine is based almost entirely on the information you give your doctor—the story you have to tell about what your headaches are like, when they began, and whether they have changed over time. What has and has not helped you in the past is crucial information for your doctor in making her diagnosis.

If you're seeing a new doctor about your headaches, she will want to obtain a complete medical history. Sometimes patients find going through the "drill" of answering questions about their past and current medical history to be tedious, even annoying, because they've already given this information to previous doctors. Why can't the new doctor just read the chart?

The fact is that each physician needs to obtain her own history rather than rely on your medical records. Your story may have changed since the last entry in your chart. Maybe you saw Dr. Lindan three years ago when your headaches were intermittent, and now they are more frequent. You've changed; medications have changed; and your new doctor will bring in a perspective that no other doctor has considered.

But probably the most important reason that your physician needs to take a new history is to uncover the material on her own. In a way, your migraine doctor is like Sherlock Holmes. The mystery of your painful headache is the conundrum that you and she will work together to solve. Your doctor will probably consider the two or three most likely possibilities, while digging for clues in your history that will allow her to discount the least likely of them.

You can help your doctor reach her goal of an accurate diagnosis by answering her questions and adding any information you think may be relevant. Like a good detective, a good doctor cannot come up with the right solution if she lacks crucial pieces of the puzzle. The information that you provide will give your doctor important clues to lead to the resolution of your own personal whodunit—in this case, why you're experiencing these headaches.

While about 85 percent of all medical diagnoses are based on a patient's medical history (with other measures such as physical examination and lab and X-ray testing contributing to the other 15 percent), with migraine, physicians place even *more* stock in medical history. Why? Because no definitive laboratory, X ray, or fingerprick blood tests exist to "prove" that your underlying problem is migraine.

However, with a thorough and exhaustive medical (and headache) history, your doctor can help make an accurate diagnosis of migraine. She'll be able to

- identify the probable cause of the headache;
- eliminate other serious diseases;
- begin to determine any headache triggers you may have;
- consider the possible impact of pregnancy, menstruation, or menopause;
- determine contributions of lifestyle or genetic factors;
- begin forming a treatment plan.

WHAT THE DOCTOR NEEDS TO KNOW

PREPARING FOR YOUR VISIT

Rather than merely responding to the questions the doctor throws at you during your appointment, take a proactive approach and write down the key points you wish to make, or the three or four questions you want to ask, during your allotted time. Although everything may seem crystal-clear to you ahead of time, it's easy to forget things in the moment or to have a conversation with a doctor take an unanticipated turn. Taking notes ahead of time will help you stay on track.

Catalog Your Symptoms
A description of your migraine symptoms is a good starting point. What is your headache pain like? Is it a tight kind of pain that feels like a constricting headband or a too-tight cap? Or is it more of a throbbing, pulsating pain? Perhaps it feels like a pressure from within. Or maybe it feels entirely different from any of these descriptions. If you have more than one type of headache, describe them all. If your head-

ache always occurs at a certain time of day or a certain time during your menstrual cycle, jot this down. (See the list of information below that the doctor needs to know.)

I'm not suggesting you write *War and Peace* or an exhaustive account of migraines and you. Bear in mind that doctors have limited time. But I do recommend hitting the high points. And since this is not English class, don't worry about crafting perfect prose. Your list might look something like this:

1. Headaches when waking up, two to three times a week
2. Pain by left eye and then to forehead
3. Which preventive med should I try?

"I make a list of three or four questions to ask my doctor, sometimes scribbled on the back of an envelope," said Joan, thirty-eight. "At our first appointment, he was a bit startled, maybe even a little apprehensive, when I pulled out my list. But now he thinks it's a super idea. He says we get a lot more information covered in our visits than he does in the same time with his other patients."

Include on your list any diagnostic procedures and tests you've already been through, and write down treatments you've already tried. If you have any reports or test results from previous doctors, bring them in. This will help your doctor gain a full picture of your headache history.

THE VISIT: THE FACTS OF THE MATTER

Between your lists, your notes, and your questions, you're extremely well prepared for your visit with your doctor. But keep in mind that especially on an initial visit, your doctor will want to do his own digging. More than likely, he'll have a whole host of questions to ask you.

MAKE HIM FEEL YOUR PAIN

The first set of questions he'll ask is likely to revolve around your pain. They may include the following:

- Where in your head does the pain occur?
- Is it always in that location, or does it vary?
- How does your headache start?
- Do you experience any kind of warning? Or do you feel well and then, all of a sudden, the pain begins?
- If there is a warning before your headache, what is it?
- Is every headache preceded by a warning?
- Are your headaches all the same, or do they vary?
- Does moving around make the pain worse?
- How long does your headache last?
- Do you have accompanying symptoms, such as nausea or vomiting?
- Do you feel a sudden need to avoid loud sounds or bright lights?
- Do you see lights or spots before your eyes?
- How often do your headaches occur?
- How long do they last?
- Do the headaches disrupt your normal activities?
- Are your menstrual cycles affected?
- If you've been pregnant, how were your migraines affected during pregnancy?

BASIC INFORMATION

Other basic information that the doctor is likely to ask during an initial examination includes the following:

- Have you had any surgeries?
- Have you had any major medical illnesses?
- Have you had any serious accidents, particularly head injuries?
- Do you have any chronic illnesses?
- What medications have you taken in the past?
- What medications do you take now?
- What medical problems do your family members experience?
- Do you smoke?

- Do you drink alcohol?
- Do you use recreational (or "street") drugs?

Answer these questions and volunteer information that seems relevant to you. Tell him about the viral meningitis that you had at age ten or the tubal ligation you had at thirty-one. Leave it up to the doctor to figure out whether this information is relevant to your headaches.

ABOUT YOUR LIFESTYLE

Because they affect your general health as well as the diagnosis and management of your headaches, personal habits like smoking and drinking are important for your doctor to know about. Information about seemingly innocuous habits such as caffeine consumption can be especially useful. If you're drinking six cans of diet soda every day, you could be unwittingly contributing to your problem. I'm not suggesting that you have to go cold turkey on caffeine (that in itself could cause a headache), but you'll want to talk to your doctor about how to reduce your caffeine consumption or cut back on other substances that might be contributing to your headaches.

Some of the questions I ask tend to surprise patients. For example, I usually ask women about their work habits, hobbies, and foreign travel. Why? Because I want to factor in the possibility of exposure to any toxins or exotic infectious diseases. I also ask about sleep patterns because they can have a significant impact on headaches.

What's more, your doctor will need to know if you use any street drugs because they could interfere with medications she might prescribe. They could also be a component in your headache pain. Many people are hesitant or fearful to provide such information, but the doctor really needs it to effectively treat your headache problem. Remember, what you tell your doctor will remain confidential.

When appropriate, it's also useful for patients to provide

specific examples of the havoc headaches wreak on their lives.

"Patients often don't say how the headache attacks are affecting their lives, and doctors are trained to focus on symptoms and diagnosis rather than the impact of the illness," writes Richard Lipton, M.D., in a 1997 article in *Headache*. However, when the patient "spells out the impact of the pain—'I'm missing two days of work every month, and I might get fired,' or 'I couldn't take care of my baby while I was sick,' " Lipton says that doctors may be even more responsive.

ALL IN THE FAMILY

The doctor will probably ask you if migraine runs in your family. You may or may not know the answer. Jodi, twenty-seven, did. "I told my doctor that migraines are a family illness. Every generation of my father's family has had people who've had what we called the 'Andrews sick headache.' But since I was diagnosed, they're finally all calling it migraine!"

If you're not sure if migraines are a family problem, ask your parents and siblings, aunts and cousins if they have been diagnosed with migraines. Also, since many migraineurs go undiagnosed, you should find out about their severe headache symptoms and patterns. Report this information to the doctor. Again, be complete. Let her be the judge of its relevance.

BRING YOUR MEDICINES TO THE APPOINTMENT

Even if you think you know what medications you're taking like the back of your hand, it's easy to forget the dosage (it happens a lot!) and sometimes even the name of the drug, especially if you're taking three or four at the same time. So although it may seem cumbersome, I always recommend that my new patients bring everything they are currently taking to their first appointment. And I mean *everything*—both prescription medications and over-the-counter ones such as decongestants or stomach remedies, vitamins, herbal supplements, aspirin, birth control pills, and even homeo-pathic treatments.

It's important to do this because medications often inter-act with one another; your doctor will need to know what's in your system in order to decide what other medications could be prescribed. Be sure to tell her about any allergies you may have. Even though the medication the doctor pre-scribes may not be the precise one to which you're allergic, some medications are sufficiently similar to cause cross-aller-gies. You can avoid this problem by providing the informa-tion up front.

Your doctor will also ask about medications you've tried in the past for your headaches or other illnesses. Which helped? Which didn't? Did any make you feel worse or cause any adverse reactions? If you've kept a list, by all means bring it in. If you've never kept a list of your medications and your reactions to them, start now.

When Rowena, thirty-six, a patient of mine who has suf-fered from migraines since she was a teenager, came to see me for the first time, she did a smart thing. She printed out a long list of drugs used in migraine therapy from the Internet and checked off the several dozen she'd tried in the past, noting their usefulness or lack thereof. I was quickly able to discern what she had never tried and prescribed one of the newer medications. It has worked wonders for her.

TAKE YOUR MEDICINE—OR TELL THE DOCTOR IF YOU WON'T (OR DON'T)

Many people either don't take their medication or don't give it a long enough trial. Experts who have studied medica-tion compliance (taking your medicine as prescribed) have found that about half of all people are not "medication-compliant." Of this group, about 20 percent don't take their medicine at all and about 30 percent are "partial compliers," which means sometimes they take it and sometimes they don't, or that they don't take it as many times a day as directed.

Why don't people take their medication as they should? There are many reasons, but the following seem to lead the pack:

- They don't think this headache will be that bad.
- They don't like the medication's side effects.
- They take a few pills and if the pain subsides think they're "cured."
- They forget.
- They can't afford to fill the prescription.

Sometimes migraine sufferers think, "Maybe this headache won't be so bad. I'll just take an aspirin and lie down." But if you do this, you may lose an opportunity to abort a migraine attack before it becomes serious. Waiting too long to take medication may mean that you'll suffer even longer. Once a migraine is fully established, it can become more difficult to reverse.

Medication compliance can also be poor when medications have annoying or uncomfortable side effects. If your medicine causes significant adverse effects, tell your doctor. She may be able to lower the dose, change the medication, combine it with another drug, or find another solution.

Do *not* wait weeks or months to tell your doctor you stopped the medication. Instead, call the office and leave a brief message for the doctor about when and why you stopped. If the doctor wants you to try something else, she will let you know.

She may also be able to change the form of the medicine if that's your reason for not taking it. If you can't take a tablet because you vomit when you have migraines, the doctor may prescribe a suppository medication or a nasal spray. Sometimes treating the nausea first, then taking the migraine medication is an effective strategy.

Another common patient error is to take medications for a few days or even a few weeks and then stop, thinking the illness has been cured. But if your medication is a preventive drug, you need to take it every day. (Read more about medications in Chapter 7.)

SHOULD YOU BE CHECKED *DURING* A MIGRAINE?

In the case of many diseases, the doctor needs to see you when you're ill in order to diagnose and treat you. But with migraine, it's not only unnecessary but could be self-defeating to show up when you're sick. While you might mistakenly assume that the doctor would be more sympathetic and understanding in the face of obvious pain and would thus work even harder to treat you, in my view, it's better to see the doctor when you can focus on your migraine and calmly and lucidly discuss your symptoms.

When your head is clear, you will also be more able to listen and respond to her suggestions for treatment. Were you in the throes of a migraine, you might miss important instructions or be unable to answer critical questions. If you're experiencing a migraine on the day of your appointment, my recommendation is to call and reschedule.

THE PHYSICAL EXAMINATION AND HEADACHE CONDITIONS

Women experience headaches for many different reasons, and the physical examination for headache enables your doctor to rule out various causes. Even if both you and your doctor are pretty well convinced that your headaches are migraines, it's possible that you are experiencing other kinds of headaches as well.

When your major complaint is headaches, your doctor (regardless of her specialty) should perform at least an abbreviated neurologic exam or should refer you to a specialist for one. This includes an examination of your eyes and facial nerves, reflexes, muscle strength, skin sensation, balance, and coordination. Because some neck conditions have been implicated as the guilty parties in some headaches, a head and neck exam may provide useful information.

HEADACHE AND THE NECK

The term "cervicogenic headache" has been used to describe a specific pattern of headache arising from bone and joint problems in the neck. A broader term of "vertebrogenic headache" has been used by chiropractors and osteopathic physicians to describe headache arising from various neck problems. It has also been noted that many patients with benign recurring headaches, both migraine and tension-type, report neck pain or will have tenderness in the neck when examined. Various disciplines (including chiropractic, osteopathic, orthopedics, and neurology) argue over the significance of all this as well as the terminology. The fact is that head and neck pain can be related, even though we do not yet fully understand all the connections in the brain.

TEMPOROMANDIBULAR HEADACHE

It's a mouthful, isn't it? In front of the ear where the jaw meets the temple is the temporomandibular joint. Abnormalities in this joint—which may arise from dental problems—can result in headache. Temporomandibular dysfunction (TMD) is sometimes treated by dentists or oral surgeons instead of, or in conjunction with, physicians. Treatment consists of medications, relaxation exercises, orthodontia, and bite splints, which are molded to your mouth by a dentist and are worn at night to prevent clenching or grinding of the teeth.

Surgery is available for treatment of severe TMD and may be appropriate for certain jaw problems. However, you should be aware that many dental professionals are concerned that TMD is overdiagnosed and overtreated. It may be wise to get a second opinion if you do not respond to conventional therapy. And you should know at the outset that jaw surgery may not relieve headache pain.

SINUS HEADACHE

If you have pain around both eyes and in the forehead, it must be a sinus headache, right? Perhaps so, but if the pain is associated with nausea, photophobia, or other typical migraine symptoms, it is actually more likely to be a migraine. Studies of headache type and frequency have shown that people with migraine often assume their headaches are sinus headaches.

Sinus headache is usually associated with mucus drainage and often with fever. If you suspect sinus headache, see your doctor. Sinusitis cannot be reliably diagnosed over the telephone; you need to be examined. You may even need a CT scan. (CT scanning of the sinuses is more accurate than an X ray or MRI scan.)

Rather than assume you have a sinus headache and treat it as such, it's best to obtain a diagnosis. Unnecessary use of antibiotics can lead to antibiotic resistance. If you've used an antibiotic and the headache hasn't gone away, it may not have been sinusitis after all. Avoid over-the-counter antihistamines or vasoconstrictive decongestants unless your doctor specifically recommends them. Use of these medications for more than three days can result in nasal congestion. It is also possible to develop rebound congestion from daily use of decongestants, especially in nasal-spray form.

STROKE

If you have no symptoms other than headache, you are probably not having a stroke. But you should know that stroke occurs in more than one variety. There are thrombotic strokes, in which a blood vessel clogs, and embolic strokes, in which a blood clot breaks off from somewhere in the body and travels in the arteries until it clogs a smaller blood vessel in the brain. Then there are small strokes, sometimes called lacunar strokes, which occur because the small blood vessels in the brain have abnormally rough linings, causing a blood clot to form on them. And there are hemorrhagic strokes, in which there is bleeding into the brain. All of these can cause headache.

The hemorrhagic type is most likely to cause headache, often associated with vomiting or neurologic deficits like numbness or paralysis (or weakness) of an arm or leg. Headaches occur in about 15 percent of thrombotic and embolic strokes. Small strokes may not cause headache, although occasionally small strokes are caused by other conditions that do cause headaches.

Stroke can occur due to migraine, though this is very rare. If you have migraine with aura, you have a slightly higher risk of stroke than does a migraineur without aura. Oral contraceptives can be a risk factor for stroke, especially in the woman who has migraine with aura. If you have an aura that lasts longer than an hour, there is an outside chance this is a stroke, so call your doctor.

BRAIN TUMORS

One of the leading anxieties of headache sufferers is that they have a brain tumor. But in reality this is very unlikely. Of all headaches experienced, less than half of 1 percent are caused by brain tumors. And only about half of all brain-tumor patients develop a headache, and that headache is likely to be mild.

In the majority of brain-tumor headache patients, the headache has characteristics similar to those of a tension-type headache (see Chapter 1). In about one-third, the headache is worse in the morning and when bending over. Migrainelike headaches have been reported in cases of brain tumor but are infrequent. One study found that only 8 percent of brain-tumor patients had headache as the *only* symptom at the time of diagnosis. However, if a headache develops for the first time over age sixty-five, there is greater likelihood it may be due to a brain tumor.

ANEURYSM/AVM

If you develop a sudden severe headache—the worst of your life, one that feels like "a bolt of lightning" or a "thunderclap headache"—and it's not quite like your usual headaches in terms of location or features, it could represent a ruptured aneurysm or arteriovenous malformation (AVM). Aneurysms are areas of thinning in the blood-vessel wall, usually caused by congenital defects in the blood vessel. Arteriovenous malformations are nests of abnormal blood vessels that you are born with. They often have abnormal walls and can have thin spots as well. Over the years, the continual pressure in the blood vessel wears the thin spot thinner, until it balloons out and begins leaking or even ruptures. The leaking of blood results in a severe headache.

If we can catch the process at this stage and intervene, we may be able to prevent damage to the brain. Often, however, we don't have this opportunity, and the aneurysm just ruptures, pouring blood into the brain and spinal fluid. Needless to say, this results in a terrible headache. Aneurysm differs from a migraine in that it usually involves the entire head. Like migraine, it may be associated with nausea, photophobia, and sonophobia, and it may involve strokelike symptoms, such as numbness or weakness on one side, or difficulty finding the words you want. However, most migraineurs do not have "focal" findings—extreme numbness or weakness, difficulty speaking, or a facial droop. If these develop for the first time in conjunction with the most severe headache you've ever had, then it's time to worry about a possible aneurysm, which can also progress to coma. In about half of cases, a warning headache occurs before rupture. This can occur days, weeks, or even months ahead of time. While it may be a severe headache, it isn't always; it just may be a different type of headache from what you're used to. If you experience an unusual headache, call your doctor. (However, if you've experienced your usual aura, followed by a unilateral headache, it's unlikely to be an aneurysmal bleed, even if the headache is severe.)

A ruptured aneurysm is a neurological emergency. If you experience a sudden severe headache unlike any you have ever had before, do not wait to see if your medication helps; take your medication and go to the emergency room. Have someone drive you, take a cab, or call 911. You can always turn around and come back home if it was a false alarm and your medication works. It's always better to be safe than sorry.

MENINGITIS AND ENCEPHALITIS

Meningitis is a viral or bacterial infection of the meninges, the lining around the brain. Headache is the most common symptom. Bacterial meningitis is a serious condition requiring hospitalization for intravenous antibiotic therapy. Patients describe the headache associated with this as severe or explosive. Fever occurs with headache in meningitis, and there is marked stiffness of the neck.

Viral meningitis is usually self-limited. There is no specific treatment for it other than pain management. It usually lasts a week or two, then spontaneously resolves itself. Lyme disease, tuberculosis, and certain fungi can also cause meningitis.

Encephalitis is an inflammation of the brain itself. It is usually viral, and it is always serious. Severe headaches often occur due to irritation of the meninges and swelling of the brain itself. (It may feel like your whole brain is swollen during a migraine, but it actually isn't.) Encephalitis is treated in the hospital with pain management and IV fluids. In some cases, encephalitis can cause a temporary coma.

CEREBROSPINAL-FLUID PRESSURE
ABNORMALITIES

Your brain is surrounded by cerebrospinal fluid (CSF), which acts like a shock absorber. Normally, our bodies make and absorb cerebrospinal fluid at the same rate, and they completely recycle it in a twenty-four-hour period. If the CSF pressure becomes too low or too high, it can cause a headache. Low-pressure syndromes are rare and occasionally occur after a diagnostic spinal tap or after you have had spinal or epidural anesthesia.

High CSF pressure can occur due to various conditions, including brain tumor, brain infection, or after a head injury with bleeding into the brain. The most common cause of high CSF pressure is a condition called "pseudotumor cerebri" or "benign intracranial hypertension." It is not clear whether this condition is the result of too much CSF production or poor absorption of CSF. We do know that the following factors are associated with its development:

- pituitary or adrenal gland disorders
- obesity
- thyroid and parathyroid gland disorders
- pregnancy
- head injury
- menstrual irregularities
- anemia
- vitamin A deficiency or overuse
- some medications (tetracycline, sulfonamides, indomethacin, phenytoin, nitrofurantoin, nalidixic acid, isotretinoin)

Benign intracranial hypertension can be treated with medication to stabilize CSF pressure.

DIAGNOSTIC TESTS

Although lab work and tests can't be the basis for migraine diagnosis, they can be useful to your doctor by ruling *out* other problems.

MRI

Your doctor may order an MRI (magnetic resonance imaging) scan, although it's not necessarily a "must-have" test. For example, if your headaches started when you were in your teens, your worst headache is with your period, you've had the same kind of headaches for twenty years, and your mother and grandmother both had similar headaches, then you probably don't need an MRI. Odds are, it's migraine.

"My mom used to get these 'sick headaches' when I was a kid, and I never understood what the big deal was," said Betsy, thirty-five. "Not until I started getting these terrible blinding headaches myself when I was around fourteen."

Sometimes an MRI is a good idea, of course. It can be useful when the doctor is worried that your headaches might be caused by a brain tumor or a blood-vessel abnormality, such as an aneurysm. Also, if it sounds to your doctor like your headaches are accompanied by unusual symptoms, or that your headache pattern has changed, he may order an MRI to make sure it's nothing serious.

What is an MRI? It's a painless imaging technology that provides physicians with an excellent picture of soft tissue (like your brain) and fluids. Brain areas of the wrong consistency could indicate swelling, bleeding, tumor development, certain kinds of infection, or other problems, such as multiple sclerosis.

Physicians can also tell if there are spots where brain-cell death has occurred, leaving a fluid-filled hole or scar. Sometimes the doctor can also see abnormal blood vessels or aneurysms on an MRI, but these do not always show clearly. For a better look, the doctor may need to order an angiogram, which is described later in this chapter.

Here's how an MRI works. The body part that the doctor is concerned about—in this case, your head—is centered in a strong magnetic field. Magnetic energy pulls the protons in your molecules out of their usual path as they spin on their axis. The time it takes for them to fall back into place is measured and turned into a picture by a computer.

What's it like to have an MRI? You lie flat on your back on a table that slides into a tunnel in the machine. (If you're claustrophobic, you may need to be sedated ahead of time.) You must lie very still, because even slight movement distorts the clarity of the picture. This caution also applies to the magnetic resonance angiogram (MRA), another test I'll describe. Sometimes contrast dye is injected into the vein to highlight areas of the brain. MRI and MRA tests can take anywhere from twenty to forty-five minutes, depending on the age of the equipment.

While the scanner is working, it often makes loud banging noises. If you end up with a migraine on the day of the test, you'll probably want to reschedule. The sounds can be grueling, especially if you're a sonophobe. Otherwise, an MRI doesn't hurt at all.

(Warning: If you have any metal implanted in your body, such as a pacemaker, you will not be able to have an MRI. The magnetic energy could not only distort the picture but could alter the settings on the pacemaker—not a risk you'll want to take.)

Orthodontic braces also make for a bad picture. Many people worry that their dental fillings could be a problem in getting an MRI, but they aren't, because none of the metals used by American dentists in fillings is magnetic.

MRA

A magnetic resonance angiogram may be used to diagnose a blood-vessel abnormality or an aneurysm. An MRA is like an MRI, but the computer is set differently to detect blood flow.

ANGIOGRAM

Occasionally, a standard "old-fashioned" angiogram may be needed to diagnose your problem. To perform an angiogram, the doctor punctures an artery in your groin and threads a catheter up into the carotid arteries in your neck. He then injects X-ray dye, called "contrast." Since the angiogram is an invasive test, it involves some risk. After hearing a description of it, most patients are not eager to undergo an angiogram. Doctors don't do this test as often as in the past, because the MRA usually can achieve much the same results.

CT SCAN

If a brain test is needed, the MRI is best because it provides the clearest picture. In some situations, however, a CT scan (short for "computer-aided tomography") may be preferable. Or the MRI might be a better choice but there's no MRI scanner in your area, especially if you live outside the United States. So the CT scan will be used instead.

A CT scan uses regular X rays but analyzes them by computer to make a picture. CT actually shows bone better than it does soft tissue. It is also very sensitive to fresh bleeding into the brain (such as in a hemorrhage). Another advantage of the CT scan is that results can be obtained slightly faster than results for MRI scans.

Other diagnostic tests your doctor may select are X rays, a CT scan of your sinuses, blood tests, or a sleep study.

SPINAL TAP

Occasionally, when infection is suspected or the CSF pressure inside your head is dangerously high, the doctor may order a diagnostic spinal tap (lumbar puncture). In this procedure, the doctor inserts a needle into your back, through the muscle layers, and into the fluid-filled space around the spinal cord. Not to worry—the needle is inserted well below where the spinal cord ends and won't injure it. The pressure of the spinal fluid is measured, and a sample of fluid is drained off for laboratory analysis. (The spinal tap can help the doctor diagnose certain diseases, such as meningitis and encephalitis.)

Your body continuously produces and absorbs spinal fluid, completely replacing your entire volume of it every twenty-four hours. So it won't hurt you to lose a little spinal fluid for analysis. Important precaution: After having a spinal tap, you should lie flat on your back and remain very still for at least four hours to prevent any possible leakage of spinal fluid. That could cause—what else?—a headache.

SLEEP STUDIES

The doctor may order a sleep study if she suspects sleep apnea or some other sleep disorder. Sleep apnea causes irregular breathing, usually associated with snoring or, dangerously, with periods when the patient briefly stops breathing.

During apnea periods, blood levels of oxygen can drop significantly, often resulting in headaches upon awakening. A sleep study is performed during the night at a clinic or hospital sleep lab. While you sleep, you wear various devices that measure your blood-oxygen levels, rate of respiration, heart rate, and brain waves.

Sleep apnea can be treated with a breathing device that you wear at night. Sometimes surgery to remove the excess tissue at the back of the throat—which generally causes snoring as well as sleep apnea—is performed for treatment.

MAKING A DIAGNOSIS

Your doctor will analyze the information obtained from his interview with you, along with a review of your records and the results of any tests he has ordered. Based on this information and his expertise and skill, he will determine your probable diagnosis. Probable? you may ask. Can't the doctor be sure? Not always, and not necessarily the first time you are seen. Instead, a "differential diagnosis" is generated.

He will rule out some diagnoses and add others as he

zeroes in on the most likely possibilities. This list changes as new pieces of information are added to the analysis, until the doctor is satisfied that he has reached the most likely diagnosis.

With your cooperation and assistance in helping him obtain the data he needs, this diagnosis will enable your doctor to form a good treatment plan to help you manage your migraines.

DO YOUR PART FOR WELLNESS

BE CANDID

Though you've shelled out the bucks, the time, and the emotional energy to consult with a doctor, you need to ask yourself: Will you try your hardest to follow your doctor's recommendations? Perhaps one of the biggest surprises for me about practicing medicine has been the degree to which patients fail to follow my advice. This is a common complaint among my physician colleagues.

"Sometimes I recommend really important things to do, and they go off and do what their Aunt Sarah's neighbor tells them to do instead," groused one physician.

Often doctors advise patients to do things they can't or won't do, such as avoiding certain foods, quitting smoking, and so forth. Try to follow your doctor's recommendations whenever possible, but be honest with yourself—and with him—and about what you're willing to try.

Consider each recommendation seriously. Tell the doctor if you feel that you can't or won't comply with one or more of them. If you don't have time for a regular exercise program, speak up. If you've tried quitting smoking but can't do it and don't wish to attempt it again, tell your doctor it's just not realistic. If you just can't give up caffeine, say so. If you've experienced serious side effects in the past from the medication that the doctor wants to prescribe, tell him this.

He may be able to prescribe a lower dose or another medication.

USING MEASURABLE MARKERS TO
EVALUATE CHANGE

Commit yourself to doing what you can and will do to aid
in your treatment. And review quantifiable markers from
your own life that you can use to help you and your doctor
evaluate your progress. To do this, identify problems related
to your migraines that may (or may not) have noticeably
improved after at least several weeks of treatment. Tracking
the frequency, duration, and severity of your migraines in a
headache diary is the primary way to do this (more on this
in Chapter 3). Other milestones, however, may help you see
how the quality of your life is improving.

Quality of life has to do with how well you are functioning. Maybe before treatment you were only able to drive your
son to kindergarten two or three days out of five and had
to ask a neighbor to drive him on the other days. But since
treatment, you feel well enough to take him most of the
time. This is a definite improvement. Or perhaps migraine
pain prevented you from working out, but now that you've
been treated you find you're as active as you want to be. Each
patient has particular benchmarks to use to judge improvement.

If you've followed your doctor's recommendations but
you're still not happy with your migraine care, the problem
may lie with your doctor.

SHOULD YOU CHANGE DOCTORS?

Perhaps you're no newcomer to medical attention for your
headaches. Or you've been working with the same physician
to manage your migraine pain for ten years. Whether you've
been working with a specialist or with a generalist, the time

may be right to evaluate whether your doctor is up to par and to determine if it's time to make a change.

If you're unhappy with the health care you're receiving for your migraines, you're not alone. A study on "perceived adequacy of care" conducted by CareData Reports in 1994 revealed that *only 34 percent* of all migraine patients rated their health care "excellent." Treatment of twenty-three health conditions—including heart disease, osteoporosis, dental care, and others—were also rated. Migraine treatment fared poorly, with only sleep problems and pain management receiving lower overall satisfaction ratings. (By contrast, 78 percent of pregnancy patients said their health care was excellent, and 60 percent of diabetes patients rated their care highly.)

While the study confirmed what I've long suspected—that many migraineurs are discontent with their care—it did not address *why* so many people were unhappy. There are a variety of possibilities, ranging from difficulties with diagnosis to a lack of adequate insurance coverage. For many, though, discontent almost certainly stems from dissatisfaction with their physician.

If you are considering changing doctors, I'll run you through the paces of how to evaluate your doctor and how to identify a good physician. Or you may be happy with your doctor but unable to obtain the specialty referral you need for migraine evaluation and treatment because of your insurance coverage. Not all doctors—otherwise good physicians—are expert in headache management. I'll recommend tactics to use with your managed-care plan to convince them you deserve appropriate care.

WHEN A CHANGE IS NEEDED

A doctor who routinely dismisses or minimizes your complaints or belittles your suffering is not the best person to be managing your migraines. For example, Doreen, forty-five, reported that the silliest—and most hurtful—comment she ever heard about her migraines came from her former physician. "The reason you have migraines is because you're afraid of sex," he told her. "If your fear of sex disappeared, then the migraines would go, too." If your doctor offers outlandish opinions like this one, rarely returns your phone calls, is hard to get an appointment with, and spends little time with you when you have one, it's definitely time to switch.

If you routinely wait until your doctor is off-duty so you can go to the emergency room instead of his office, take this as a strong signal that you need to consider changing physicians. If you find yourself doubling over in pain from migraine time and again, but *not* calling your doctor because you know nothing will happen anyway, clearly a change is in order.

THREE COMMON PHYSICIAN PROBLEMS

There are three primary problems that are surprisingly common among physicians who treat migraine. The first is the doctor who simply isn't knowledgeable about migraines. This type of physician often prescribes only pain pills rather than migraine-specific medications or preventative medications.

A second major problem is that many physicians have an attitude about migraines. They do not take the problem seriously and fall into the dismissive "it's-only-a-headache" group that you've doubtless encountered in the general population. Some of these physicians are reluctant to prescribe medications to women with migraine, either because they feel medication is unnecessary or because they perceive that narcotics are required, and they disapprove of narcotics or have concerns about prescribing them on an ongoing basis.

The third major problem has less to do with migraine expertise and more with patient care in general. It is the physician who is not willing to partner with you in determining the best care or who seems too busy to give your migraine problem sufficient attention—even if your physician is knowledgeable about headaches.

I'll give you my thumbnail analysis of each of these three common problems. As you read them, ask yourself if you see your current doctor in any of these scenarios.

Just Because He's a Doctor Doesn't Mean He's Migraine-Savvy

Graduation from medical school and an M.D. license do not automatically guarantee detailed knowledge of migraine. In many medical schools, headaches are covered primarily as a symptom of other diseases, and only scant information regarding migraine is taught. In addition, research in the field of migraine is advancing very rapidly, with new things being discovered all the time. Doctors need to keep up with a changing medical world. While it's a challenge for specialists to stay abreast of new advances in their fields, it's almost impossible for primary-care physicians to keep up with advances in everything.

While a physician specializing in neurology is generally a good bet to treat your migraine, not all neurologists are equally knowledgeable. Some have chosen subspecialties within the field, such as stroke, multiple sclerosis, and epilepsy, and choose to focus primarily on those.

In nearly all cases, your best choice is a doctor who runs a headache clinic. A physician who cares enough about headache to dedicate his entire practice to it is likely to take your migraines very seriously.

Attitude Is Important

If the physician stereotypes women with migraines as whiners and babies or suspects migraineurs of making up excuses to obtain narcotics, look for a different doctor.

Susan, forty-one, has experienced migraines for years and confided that previous doctors treated her "either like a child or a junkie in search of a fix. They didn't seem to understand what was at stake: that I had to continue to function or I'd lose my job." An astute physician can offer appropriate migraine treatment and can usually readily detect the drug-seeking patient within the first few visits.

Fear of Drugs

Many physicians are reluctant to prescribe strong medications, particularly narcotics, for fear they will be sanctioned for prescribing "too many" drugs. Or they may worry that a patient could become psychologically or physically dependent on them.

These medication concerns are valid; however, it's equally valid to consider the severity of your pain and the frequency of your attacks. If the physician is so loath to prescribe strong medications that you suffer as a result, it's time to consider switching doctors.

Darla, twenty-four, is an example. She told me that at first her family doctor didn't believe her migraines were severe. Instead, she tried to convince her that they weren't so bad. One day Darla had an attack during an office visit. She was so clearly suffering that her doctor finally knew how sick she was.

"Now she believes I'm in pain and will reluctantly prescribe for me," says Darla. "But my problem is that she doesn't like the medications I'm on because of her beliefs that women of childbearing age shouldn't take meds that could be harmful to a possible pregnancy."

Darla's migraines can be so severe that in the past she actually contemplated suicide when she was denied medication. "I would pray I would pass out so the pain would go away," she said. Now that her doctor is grudgingly prescribing medication, Darla feels she's regained some control, although she still feels guilty, knowing her doctor disapproves of migraine medications. Darla should consider changing doctors.

The "Now Just Relax, Dear" Syndrome

The patronizing attitude that some physicians—male and female—demonstrate toward women is tough to stomach.

April, thirty-four, a migraine patient for years, told me, "I had one doctor who discounted the whole problem as a 'woman thing.' I'd been in chronic pain for months, and he downplayed it and wouldn't order a single test or refer me to a neurologist."

April decided to take charge. "I fired him and got a new primary-care doc who quickly approved a neurological consult and an MRI," she said. "This proved to me that it's not so much the system that's a problem, but it's how hard your doctor works for you and how willing you are to compliantly accept what is dished out to you."

It may surprise you to know that the prejudice against migraine in some quarters of the medical community is not exclusive to women. I've been surprised to hear from several male migraineurs that they, too, have dealt with doctors who were unsympathetic—even contemptuous—of their pain.

Bill, forty-one, said that when a doctor once told him, "It's only a headache!" he felt like "beating him in the head with a bat and saying, 'But doctor, it's *only* a severe beating!' "

SHOULD YOU CHANGE DOCTORS?
KEY QUESTIONS

Here's a short self-test to help you decide whether you should change physicians. Answer "yes" or "no" to each question:

	Yes	No
1. If you experience more than two migraines per week, have you been offered preventative medications?	☐	☐
2. Have you asked your doctor for a migraine-specific medication and been denied without an explanation being offered?	☐	☐

	Yes	No
3. Has your doctor ever said to you, "But it's *only* a headache."	☐	☐
4. If you run out of medication unexpectedly, can you get a prescription refill from your doctor within twenty-four hours?	☐	☐
5. Does your doctor offer only narcotics, muscle relaxants, or sedating medications, rather than migraine-specific medications?	☐	☐
6. When you ask your doctor about new medications that you've heard about, does she say that she doesn't know or have time to learn about them?	☐	☐

If you answered "yes" to more than three questions, it's time for you to start looking for a new physician.

FINDING A NEW PHYSICIAN

You've decided you do need a new doctor. How do you find a good one? There are a number of important considerations—not the least of which is your health care plan. If you're one of many Americans under a managed-care plan today, that means you can't go to any doctor you feel like whenever you feel like it—at least, not if you want the insurance company to pick up all or part of the tab.

While there are too many medical plans for me to describe each one, virtually all plans provide some choice. For example, even though you have one primary-care provider to manage your overall health care, usually you can select that person from a pool of approved doctors. Ask an employee at the health care plan for a list of approved doctors and specialists in your area. To track down the best doctor for you, consider the following pointers.

- Ask your friends and neighbors if they've heard of any of the doctors on the list. If a friend gives you an opinion, ask why she likes Dr. Dombrowski but doesn't care for Dr. Stern. But keep in mind that the doctor your best friend likes may not be ideal for you.

- Quiz any other doctors you know—even your gynecologist or dermatologist—for a recommendation of doctors on the list. An acquaintance of mine received a recommendation from her child's pediatrician for a highly effective internist, one she has been with for years.

- Whenever possible, try to set up a telephone "preinterview" with the physician you're considering. (It's not always possible to get through, but if you do, limit the time you take to three to five minutes.) Avoid launching into a description of your symptoms, and don't try to pump him for free advice. A physician can't give you advice without first examining you. Instead, use your time to ask the doctor if he treats many migraine patients and how he usually treats migraines.

- If you can't interview the doctor over the phone, talk to her nurse to find out how often she treats migraine; the more experienced the doctor is with migraines, the better off you're likely to be.

- Is the physician a member of the American Council for Headache Education or the National Headache Foundation? It's not necessary that a good doctor be a member of either group, but membership is a clear indication that he's interested in migraines.

- If possible—even if you have to pay for it out of your own pocketbook—see the doctor in person. Personal interaction with the doctor will give you an idea of whether this is the person to whom you want to entrust your health.

GOING OUTSIDE THE MANAGED-CARE SYSTEM

Here's a tough dilemma for those under managed care. What if you can't find a doctor you like within the pool of approved doctors your plan offers? And you're not able to change your plan or your primary physician? Should you see someone outside the system?

First, find out if your managed-care company will pay a physician outside its preferred-provider list. Most do not advertise this feature, but they may pay for an "out-of-network" doctor. (If they do, they'll probably pay at a lower rate than for a doctor in the system. This is sometimes called a "point-of-service" option.)

Suppose you want to see a neurologist, and your family doctor agrees that this is a good idea. But the specialist is not on your plan's list of approved doctors. Ask your doctor to write a justification for you to be examined by a doctor outside the regular system. Although physicians complain that nobody ever listens to them, the fact of the matter is that the insurance company is more likely to pay attention if a doctor says that you need to see another doctor in another city than if you tell them the same thing.

If this tactic doesn't work, try to think of a way that seeing that new doctor would be cost-effective for the insurance company, and put it in writing. Find out the name of the supervisor of your insurance company's claims department and address your letter to that person.

Opposite is a sample letter that I invite you to adapt to your own situation. I can't guarantee it'll work, but it's worth a try. Be sure to include your name, your daytime phone number, and your policy number in the letter.

You may also be able to make headway through telephone calls. However, be sure to get the name of the person you talked to, and always follow up with a letter summarizing the agreement you've made. It's good to have a paper trail when dealing with insurance companies.

PROPER TREATMENT CUTS COSTS

The authors of an article in a 1998 issue of *The American Journal of Managed Care* compared the medical expenses of a

SAMPLE LETTER

55 Laurel Lane
Peoria, IL 60000
Tel: (555) 444-3333
Oct. 15, 1999

Ms. Clementine Clout
Purple Cross Insurance Company
47 Elm St.
Anywhere, IL 60000

Dear Ms. Clout:

I need your assistance in obtaining permission to see a doctor outside the insurance pool network who can help me with my migraine headaches. I am employed and insured by the Acme Widget Company. My policy number is 897-345-987. I have located a doctor I want to see. If you approve this request, it will save your company a considerable amount of money and could put an end to my debilitating pain.

I have suffered from severe migraine headaches for ten years now. They've gotten so bad that I've missed many work days and much time with my family. My family doctor, Dr. Carlton Kerley, has tried to help me but to no avail. He thinks I need to see a specialist. The two neurologists I've called on your approved list are booked up for six months.

I need immediate help. I located Dr. Margo MacKnight at the Happy Headache Clinic here in town, and she can see me within two weeks. But I need your approval to pay for the visit. I understand that, if approved, you would pay at the 80 percent rate rather than the 90 percent rate.

How will approving my request save your company money? Because I have had to go to the emergency room eight times in the past six months for migraines. Each emergency room visit costs over $400, so the tab has already added up to over $3,200 this year alone.

If I can see Dr. MacKnight, she can advise me and prescribe the right medication. Dr. MacKnight told me that anybody who has as many migraines as I do needs an evaluation. If she's right, a lot of dollars will be saved, and my pain will be alleviated.

Thanks in advance for considering my request. I look forward to your prompt and positive decision.

Sincerely,
Sally N. Payne

twenty-six-year-old woman with migraines, both before and after her visits to a headache clinic. The total medical expenses for her headaches before seeing the headache specialist included physician fees, emergency-room visits, and medication, and came to nearly $3,900 per year. After seeing the specialist, the woman's annual medical expenses plummeted to around $1,200—less than one-third of the expenses previously incurred.

The article summarizes the point I've long made, both to insurance companies and managed-care officials, as well as to prospective patients: "Specialists in headache centers are better able to accurately and rapidly arrive at correct diagnoses and address and reinforce issues of headache education than busy generalists."

WHAT IF YOUR INSURANCE COMPANY JUST SAYS NO?

What if your insurance company fails to be persuaded by logic? My advice to patients is to never give up. Call Ms. Clout and tell her you plan to appeal her decision. Then do it. Virtually every insurance company has some sort of appeals process. And almost every person in Ms. Clout's position hates it when someone appeals.

Why? Because appeals mean more paperwork, writing reports, and having someone else review her work— someone with the authority to overrule her decision. She might change her mind, right then and there while you are on the phone, when you say the word *appeal*. If she still says no, do appeal. Often you can appeal two or more times. Each time, a person at a higher level must review your appeal. Many appeals succeed.

One cautionary note: Sometimes nothing you do works. If you're turned down, your appeals fail, and you're still miserable, what should you do?

First of all, never underestimate the value of a strong emotional appeal. Tell Dr. Kerley that he has been a wonderful doctor to you but this migraine problem is making you crazy and maybe this other doctor, Dr. MacKnight, whose complete expertise is headaches, has an idea that could work. You might be able to convince your regular doctor to order the tests that the headache clinic doctor wants run, or even to prescribe medications based on the headache specialist's recommendations.

Then tell the headache doctor that you've pulled out all the stops but your recalcitrant insurance company refuses to budge and authorize a visit. Tell her you don't think you could afford expensive tests but you'd like to at least see her to find out if she has any ideas for you.

STAND UP FOR YOUR HEALTH

The main point to keep in mind when deciding whether to find another doctor is that your health—not the doctor's feelings—should be your paramount concern.

If you've taken my self-test and your physician does *not* measure up, it's time for a change. My guess is that after you've found a new, sympathetic, and capable doctor, you'll wonder why you wasted all that time with your former physician.

Becky, fifty-four, after years of enduring inadequate care for her migraines at last has found the kind of treatment she needs. She told me, "For the first thirty years of migraines, my doctors did not understand my problem. They thought my migraines had come about because I was an only child or wanted attention or because I was a young woman. Now I have a really great neurologist whose wife and adult son both have migraines. He even set up a migraine support group. He's terrific, and I can't begin to describe the difference he's made in my life."

If you do your homework and track down the best physician for you, and if you work with your doctor as a partner in pain management, my belief is that you, like Becky, can also find real relief for your migraines.

CHAPTER

3

❖

Migraine Triggers and What to Do About Them

So far, you've learned what migraine is and how to work with a doctor to manage your pain. But out there every day in the real world, you battle not only the factors that may trigger your headaches but erroneous perceptions that can give your ego and self-esteem a battering. I'll review the major migraine triggers and give you advice on how to identify them in yourself and prevent the onset of—or mitigate—a migraine attack.

MIGRAINE TRIGGERS

Since we've already debunked the common myths surrounding migraine in Chapter 1, the next step for you is determining how to avoid migraine attacks as much as possible. The best way to accomplish this is to learn about the various triggers that can bring a migraine on. In fact, the closest thing most of us have to "cause and effect" when dealing with migraines are our headache triggers.

WHAT IS A MIGRAINE TRIGGER?

A migraine trigger is a thing, action, or situation that sets into motion a chain of events that ends in a migraine.

Migraines are triggered by many things including changes in the weather, a menstrual period, a sudden shift in stress level, alterations in daily routine, or a particular odor or food. Many migraineurs report that high ambient temperatures bother them, while others say that dehydration makes them more prone to these agonizing headaches.

It's important to understand that triggers do not *cause* migraines. A trigger cannot induce migraines unless you're already predisposed to experiencing them. Migraine is a reaction to both internal (neurochemical) events and external (environmental) events. A trigger can set off either. Bear in mind that triggers are not universal; what sets off a migraine attack in one person might have no effect on you whatsoever. Identifying and understanding your personal migraine triggers is crucial because the more patterns you can identify in your migraine occurrences, the more likely you'll be to avoid at least some of them.

TRIGGER-HAPPY: THE MORE, THE MIGHTIER

Let's look at Carolyn, a migraineur who, when she encountered several triggers in combination, succumbed to a wrenching attack. The day she entered the restaurant for a big company luncheon, she was already stressed-out and in a foul mood because of problems at work. Everyone there was having a glass of red wine and invited her to join them. She was looking for a little relief and also didn't want to seem prudish, so—what the heck!—she had one, too. The restaurant was brightly lit with fluorescent lights. Some of the people in her group were smoking, and Carolyn was seated next to a coworker who positively reeked of perfume. The next thing she knew, Carolyn had come down with a nasty migraine.

What caused it? Was it the stress, her mood, the wine, the lights, the smoke, the perfume—or was it something else altogether? More than likely it was all the above triggers in combination. It's not clear in Carolyn's case which triggers were the most bothersome, but one thing is certain: Migraine triggers are *additive*. If you're susceptible to several triggers, experiencing two or more simultaneously makes you far more likely to develop a migraine than experiencing one in isolation. Some women are susceptible to a given trigger only when encountered in conjunction with another.

This doesn't mean that Carolyn should throw up her hands in despair or resolve to be a party pooper from now on. Many of her triggers were avoidable. She could have worked to clear her mind of stressful thoughts before coming to the party, refused the red wine (or merely taken a social sip or two), and carefully selected a seat away from the smoker and perfumed partier. Keeping a migraine diary would help Carolyn learn to which triggers she is most susceptible.

YOUR MIGRAINE DIARY

Keeping a migraine diary will help you take control of your life and better cope with your predisposition toward these menacing headaches. If you're not aware of your personal migraine triggers, this tool will help you—and your doctor— become more attuned. I recommend that all my patients keep one. Your migraine diary will enable you to track your own patterns and be your own detective in determining what your headache triggers may be.

I suggest that you photocopy the Women's Headache Diary and faithfully make entries every day for at least four weeks, preferably for two to three months. Why so long? You need to collect sufficient data because your migraine patterns may not be immediately apparent. When you're under stress or if you're in contact with something that triggers migraine for you, your brain doesn't always react right away. Sometimes the migraine can take hours, even days, to occur. Occasionally, the delay is even longer. Tracking your responses over time in the Women's Headache Diary can help you identify these patterns.

I have carefully selected the most salient factors in women who experience migraines, including hours of sleep, regularity of meals, possible food triggers, stress and mood changes, weather changes, and other factors. If you're still menstruating, note the date your period starts and stops in the "Comments" section at the bottom of the diary. Track when your headaches occur, how long they last, how bad they are, and what's going on at the time. Record what foods you ate that might have served as triggers. Note whether you skipped a meal, slept poorly, were under stress, or whether the Santa Ana winds came gusting in that night. It may take a while to identify a pattern, but once you discover that a migraine occurs every time you eat an avocado, it'll be relatively easy to avoid that trigger. Or you may learn that you get a migraine whenever the weather changes, or when you skip lunch. Or that red wine is a major headache trigger for you. Perhaps migraine is a problem because you slept only five hours, as opposed to your usual eight. Whatever the case, the migraine diary should help you determine your particular problems and patterns.

Once you identify your own headache patterns, you will be greatly empowered. Bring the diary with you to your next doctor's appointment, so you can go over the chart with your physician. She may see patterns and be able to make recommendations that help control the number of migraines you experience.

Remember, this is a tool for you, so adapt it to your own needs. Use the additional space on the bottom to make notes. Try to record your information on the day it happens. It's too easy to forget what happened yesterday and, consequently, to miss important and useful information that can help you discern patterns in your own headache care.

FOURTEEN TRIGGERS

Below is a list of fourteen of the most common migraine triggers, followed by an in-depth description of each, along with

WOMEN'S WEEKLY MIGRAINE DIARY

Start Date: _____

	Headache Started	Headache Stopped	Headache Severity	Stress Level	Hours Sleep Last Night	Mood	Possible Food Triggers	Recent Weather Changes?	Acute Migraine Meds: Time to Relief?	Acute Migraine Meds: Degree of Relief?
SUNDAY	Awoke With Morning Afternoon Evening	No Headache Morning Afternoon Evening	0 None 1 Mild 2 Moderate 3 Severe	Low Medium High	0–3 Hours 4–5 Hours 6–7 Hours 8+ Hours	Negative Neutral Positive		Yes No		None Mild Moderate Headache Free
MONDAY	Awoke With Morning Afternoon Evening	No Headache Morning Afternoon Evening	0 None 1 Mild 2 Moderate 3 Severe	Low Medium High	0–3 Hours 4–5 Hours 6–7 Hours 8+ Hours	Negative Neutral Positive		Yes No		None Mild Moderate Headache Free
TUESDAY	Awoke With Morning Afternoon Evening	No Headache Morning Afternoon Evening	0 None 1 Mild 2 Moderate 3 Severe	Low Medium High	0–3 Hours 4–5 Hours 6–7 Hours 8+ Hours	Negative Neutral Positive		Yes No		None Mild Moderate Headache Free
WEDNESDAY	Awoke With Morning Afternoon Evening	No Headache Morning Afternoon Evening	0 None 1 Mild 2 Moderate 3 Severe	Low Medium High	0–3 Hours 4–5 Hours 6–7 Hours 8+ Hours	Negative Neutral Positive		Yes No		None Mild Moderate Headache Free
THURSDAY	Awoke With Morning Afternoon Evening	No Headache Morning Afternoon Evening	0 None 1 Mild 2 Moderate 3 Severe	Low Medium High	0–3 Hours 4–5 Hours 6–7 Hours 8+ Hours	Negative Neutral Positive		Yes No		None Mild Moderate Headache Free
FRIDAY	Awoke With Morning Afternoon Evening	No Headache Morning Afternoon Evening	0 None 1 Mild 2 Moderate 3 Severe	Low Medium High	0–3 Hours 4–5 Hours 6–7 Hours 8+ Hours	Negative Neutral Positive		Yes No		None Mild Moderate Headache Free
SATURDAY	Awoke With Morning Afternoon Evening	No Headache Morning Afternoon Evening	0 None 1 Mild 2 Moderate 3 Severe	Low Medium High	0–3 Hours 4–5 Hours 6–7 Hours 8+ Hours	Negative Neutral Positive		Yes No		None Mild Moderate Headache Free

Note: If Menstruating Enter Start Date: _____ and End Date: _____

Comments

tips to help you avoid these triggers and thus a side-splitting headache.

1. stress
2. fatigue/lack of sleep
3. travel
4. weather changes
5. bright lights/glare
6. loud sounds
7. chemicals
8. odors
9. smoking
10. foods
11. food additives
12. skipping meals
13. caffeine withdrawal
14. alcohol

1. Stress

A dramatic change in your stress level is a leading migraine trigger. Like a car braking from fifty-five to five miles an hour in a matter of seconds, suddenly going from high stress to no stress is far more taxing on your system's equilibrium than gradually downshifting your stress level. Migraine attacks do not necessarily occur at the time of stress; delayed reactions are fairly common, with migraines often occurring hours later or even the following day.

Obviously, stress cannot always be avoided. But there is much you can do to minimize stress in your life. Try not to overschedule your life, and remember to pace yourself. Take breaks—even if they're only for five minutes—and change your posture and activity, and even the scenery, whenever possible. Alternate tasks that demand concentration with those that require something more physical, like running errands or rearranging stock. And when the stress of the moment is over, try to pamper yourself. When combined with other triggers, stress makes migraine more likely to occur.

I do want to draw one important distinction here. Many people who think they're under chronic stress may actually be depressed. And as I've said before, depression is more common among migraineurs than among the general population.

So how do you know if you're depressed? Acute depression is often obvious. You're down or sad, and it's difficult to feel happy—even if nothing is obviously wrong at the time. But chronic depression is less apparent. If you've been living in a chronically stressed state for some time, you may have become desensitized to it. Here are some of its symptoms:

- difficulty sleeping
- lack of appetite or increased eating, especially of high-fat, high-carbohydrate "comfort" foods
- feeling that nothing seems fun anymore—even things you used to enjoy
- lack of sex drive
- low energy level
- feelings of hopelessness
- tendency to cry more easily than usual
- irritability
- losing things frequently
- feeling overwhelmed by your situation both at work and at home and like you're on a treadmill

If you see yourself in this list and suspect that you may be depressed, talk to your doctor about it. Medication and counseling can usually bring a depression problem under control and make your life more enjoyable.

2. Fatigue/Lack of Sleep
Lack of sleep can be a significant factor in the frequency and severity of the migraines. Many migraineurs that I see in my practice are not initially aware that they are sleep-deprived; they assume that the six hours of sleep they get each night

are adequate. With further questioning, however, many report that their sleep is not restorative—they still feel tired in the morning. I have tracked sleep patterns in all the headache patients I've seen in the last four years. About two-thirds report nonrestorative sleep, with difficulty falling asleep or with staying asleep (or both) as a symptom. If you suspect that sleep deprivation might be a trigger for you, try getting more sleep. At the same time, work to make sure your bedtime is fairly consistent.

Sleeping in on weekends several hours later than usual is another clear-cut migraine trigger. If you get up every weekday at seven o'clock, resist the temptation to sleep till noon (or even ten o'clock) on Saturday. It's best to arise within one hour of your usual time if you find that sleeping in brings on your migraine. Likewise, avoid staying up half the night and partying if morning-after fatigue serves as a trigger for you.

If, after following these suggestions, you continue to find your sleep to be nonrestorative, you may wish to discuss the possibility of undergoing a sleep study with your physician. This is especially relevant if you snore. You might have a sleep disorder, such as sleep apnea, which can increase the frequency of your migraines.

3. Travel

Travel can be a migraine trigger no matter what your mode of transportation, but airplane travel is especially implicated. Many factors can contribute to a migraine: the stress of getting to the airport in time for the flight; the confusion, commotion, noise, lights, and odors of a crowded airport; the air-pressure changes involved in flight; dietary changes or skipped meals; and the dehydration that often occurs.

Crossing time zones—especially from west to east—can be a trigger as well. I find that I am more susceptible to a migraine attack when I fly to the East Coast from the Northwest. Yet I can fly for several hours north or south and not feel the slightest twinge of a symptom. (Fortunately, medication—both preventative and for acute treatment of migraine—has helped me resolve my transcontinental-flight problem.)

To minimize the impact of travel-induced migraine, drink lots of fluids—especially on long flights—and avoid alcohol, which is dehydrating. If you're delayed because of weather, you may not have time to dine between flights, and if there's turbulence, food and beverage service may be curtailed or even canceled. So I recommend tucking your own bottled water or juice and snacks into your carry-on bag for easy access.

Be sure to bring your migraine medication with you onto the plane. The National Headache Foundation recommends that you carry about twice as much headache medicine as you normally need when traveling, just in case. And try to remember a few days before you leave to check to make certain you have an adequate supply so that you won't add the anxiety of needing a last-minute refill to your other travel stresses.

4. Weather Changes

While there's not much you can do about the weather except complain about it, you should know that weather changes are a surprisingly common migraine trigger in women. One recent study showed that weather changes precipitated migraines in 47 percent of the women.

If you have identified a weather-sensitive pattern in yourself, you may want to stay on top of any weather changes by keeping a close eye on the news so you can anticipate fronts moving into your area.

Many weather-related migraines are triggered by barometric-pressure changes, while extreme heat or cold temperatures bring on others. If your migraines are triggered by heat, you can gain some control by remaining in an air-conditioned environment and by drinking lots of water and juice. If you're triggered by cold weather, wear appropriate cold-weather gear when going outdoors. (Silk stockings and underwear add a lot of protection without much bulk.) Your headache diary can help you determine your degree of weather sensitivity.

5. *Bright Lights/Glare*

Flickering fluorescent lighting can be a migraine trigger. Try changing the ballast in the fixture to eliminate the flickering; if you still find fluorescent lighting to be troublesome, turn off the overheads and illuminate your desk or workstation with a conventional table lamp. (This may not be possible in all work environments.)

If you're sensitive to glare, remember that glare can occur even on a cloudy day, especially if there is snow on the ground or if you're near the water. Try to carry sunglasses with you everywhere you go, and remember to put them on before you step out into the sunshine.

Alternating patterns of light and shade—such as sunlight shining through trees—can also trigger a migraine, as can strobe or randomly flashing lights. Whenever possible, avoid these triggers. Try to curtail driving at sunset or sunrise. Likewise, whenever possible, avoid driving at night so you won't be confronted with the glare of oncoming headlights.

6. *Snap, Crackle, Pop*

Sound triggers migraines less frequently than light and glare. When sound is a trigger, there usually has to be a fairly significant amount of noise—either a very loud sound or a continuous disorganized sound, such as the din of a crowd or a rock concert.

Obviously the best antidote to this trigger is to avoid the noise. If you're unable to do this, try wearing earplugs; carry a pair with you at all times. If you work in a noisy environment and don't need to interact with others or the public, headphones can provide you with classical music or other soothing sounds. A colleague with migraine who travels periodically to New York has found the night noises in the city to be so troublesome that she has a hard time sleeping at her hotel (and invariably develops a migraine the following morning). Luckily, she's found a solution. She now packs a "white noise" machine that fills her temporary quarters with the peaceful sounds of waves pounding the shore and sea-gulls calling.

7. Chemicals

A number of chemicals can trigger migraine. Some common household triggers include kerosene and naphthalene (sometimes used in mothballs and found on clothes that have been dry-cleaned). Other chemicals that trigger migraine are most frequently encountered in industrial or professional settings. When Olivia-Sophia, twenty-eight, drew a connection between the desk cleaner used by the custodial staff at her office and her migraines and asked that they stop cleaning her desk with the stuff, she was able to eliminate one workplace trigger.

Because chemicals are more likely to affect you if you're in an enclosed space (which serves to concentrate the vapors), when solvents have been used around your house you may find some relief by stepping outside and/or opening the windows to air out the room. If garden pesticides are a trigger for you, mix them in a well-ventilated space, or buy them premixed or use a natural alternative. Lauren, a thirty-seven-year-old migraineur who's triggered by chemical fertilizers and weed killers, reported that when she assigned her teenage son to handle the lawn care, her incidence of migraine dropped significantly.

If you use chemicals in the workplace and suspect they may be triggering your headaches, ask to see the MSDS (Material Safety Data Sheet). The Occupational Health and Safety Administration (OSHA) requires that this information be made available to all employees upon request. If headaches are listed as a side effect and you regularly work with a particular chemical, you may need to work under an exhaust hood or to wear a respirator.

Occasionally, formalin or formaldehyde are used in the finishing process for fabric, usually heavier fabrics like those used for upholstery or home decor. If the fabric is washable, prewashing before sewing can remove most of the chemical odor.

8. Odors

Odors are common triggers for many migraineurs. Some are very sensitive to perfumes. Highly complex perfumes with many aromatic components tend to pose the biggest problem, along with heavy, spicy perfumes. I avoid wearing most perfumes to the office, as I would hate to trigger someone's migraine. But when I am in a perfume mood, I dab on Vanilla Musk. I've worn it for two years now and have never had a complaint. Light floral, woodsy, or fruity perfumes are usually tolerated best. Try to avoid perfume-spraying salespeople at the entrance of department stores; you never know what they'll lay on you.

Incense can often trigger a migraine. For that reason, import or bath shops can prove problematic because of the incense, soap, and candle odors all attacking your senses at once. If you need something, order by catalog or send a friend in to purchase an item for you.

Gasoline can occasionally trigger migraines. If you find that to be true for you, it's definitely worth paying a few extra cents per gallon to have someone else pump your gas for you. (In Oregon this is never a problem, since my state has outlawed self-serve gas pumps.)

Cigarette smoke is a frequent migraine trigger. I once had a transcriptionist who was a heavy smoker. If those smoke-saturated reports landed on my desk right before lunch, it was a guaranteed migraine for me. Pipe-tobacco smoke is seldom as strong a trigger as the smoke from cigarettes and cigars. And wood smoke is much less likely to be a trigger than cigarette or cigar smoke.

9. Smoking

Smoking is itself a migraine trigger, and not just from exposure to the odor. Cigarettes have a number of chemical components that may have various effects. In particular, nicotine can alter the reactivity of blood vessels, triggering migraine. In heavy smokers, carbon monoxide in the blood may reach high enough levels to trigger a headache.

If you're a smoker who suffers from migraines, my best advice to you is to quit now. Over-the-counter nicotine-cessation products, like gums and patches, can help, but if they aren't enough to do the trick, your doctor may be able to help with prescription medications that can stop the craving.

Passive smoke inhalation can also be a major headache trigger. If you live with a smoker who can't or won't quit, set some guidelines to protect your health. Ask that person to smoke outside your home or in closed, designated areas in the house, which you can avoid.

10. Foods

Following is a list of foods that can serve as migraine triggers. I am not suggesting that you cut each and every one out of your diet. Rather, I would like you to be aware that they are potential migraine triggers. When you eat them, pay special attention to their effect on you over the next forty-eight hours and note it in your migraine diary.

CHOCOLATE. This trigger gets a lot of press. In fact, most migraineurs *are* able to eat chocolate without disastrous results. Dawn Marcus, M.D., and her research team at the University of Pittsburgh compared chocolate with carob in a double-blind study published in 1997. No difference was found in the number of migraines that occurred in the chocolate or in the carob groups, even among the migraineurs who believed chocolate was a trigger for them.

What's more, some migraineurs actually report headache *relief* from chocolate. Because chocolate is a highly complex food from a biochemical perspective, I'm not surprised that it can have either a positive or negative effect. What's more, you should be aware that chocolate does *not* contain caffeine but does contain a chemical called theobromine, which is in the same family as caffeine. You would have to eat a lot of chocolate to equal the amount of caffeine in a cup of coffee. (See more on caffeine withdrawal in the next section.)

AGED CHEESE. The usual suspects in this category are anything with blue or green veins—Roquefort, Stilton, and others. Sharp aged Cheddar can sometimes be a trigger. Softer cheeses are generally less aged and are less likely to be triggers.

FERMENTED DAIRY PRODUCTS. Sour cream, buttermilk, and yogurt can be migraine triggers but somewhat less often than the aged cheeses.

CITRUS. Citrus fruits and juices are moderately common as a migraine trigger. Some migraineurs react only to one citrus—usually oranges or grapefruit; others react to any citrus fruit. However, you'd need to take a bite or drink some juice; a mere twist of lemon in your iced tea isn't likely to trigger a migraine.

NUTS. These are a relatively infrequent trigger. Sometimes one type of nut, such as walnuts or pecans, can trigger your migraine; occasionally, it is the most commonly available nuts like peanuts that will do the trick.

LEGUMES. This category includes peas, beans, and soy products. Italian broad beans (or fava beans) are especially likely to be a trigger. It takes focused attention to your diet and headache diary to determine if legumes are indeed a trigger for you. If you find that they are, you'll have to be vigilant in avoiding them because soybean products especially are extremely popular and found in many dishes.

Sherine, one of my headache patients, was having about twenty headache days a month, despite being on two preventative medications for migraine. After reading that legumes could cause migraines, she has, with difficulty, eliminated peas, beans, soy products, and peanuts from her diet.

Sherine's migraine frequency has been cut in half; she now suffers about ten headache days per month.

ONIONS/GARLIC. Onions and garlic are triggers of moderate frequency among migraineurs. Some patients report that raw onions are more likely to be a problem than cooked onions; others note no difference. As with legumes, if you find onions and/or garlic to be a trigger, you'll need to be watchful because they crop up frequently in restaurant food, especially in ethnic, vegetarian, and exotic establishments.

BANANAS. Bananas are a moderately frequent trigger in women with migraine. Several of my patients report that they must avoid bananas when they are otherwise susceptible to migraine, particularly when they are premenstrual.

PINEAPPLE. Fresh or dried pineapple occasionally serves as a migraine trigger.

PAPAYA. Infrequently, papaya brings about migraines.

FIGS. Figs can trigger migraines in a small number of women. Preserved or dried figs tend to be more of a problem than fresh figs.

PICKLED FOODS. The pickled food most commonly reported as a migraine trigger is pickled herring. Sauerkraut can also turn a nasty trick. And while dill and sweet pickles can trigger a headache, the majority of migraineurs are not affected by them.

AVOCADOS. Occasionally, avocados act as a migraine trigger.

OLIVES. Olives are an infrequent trigger.

YEASTY FOODS. Foods high in yeast, such as freshly baked bread, occasionally trigger a migraine.

Food Additives

MSG. MSG is a fairly common trigger. While many migraineurs know to ask for Chinese food without MSG, most do not know that salad-bar greens are often treated with MSG to keep them fresh and green. When eating at a salad bar, ask your waiter or the manager if the salad materials have been treated with MSG. Be aware that MSG can also be found in packaged foods, especially sauce and gravy mixes. It pays to read labels.

NITRATES/NITRITES. Nitrites are used to preserve meats such as hot dogs, bologna and other luncheon meats, bacon, salami, and other hard sausages. Nitrates can also form in vegetables left in the refrigerator too long. My advice is, if it isn't crisp, toss it out. These chemicals, whether added to food or naturally developed, can trigger migraines.

ASPARTAME. This artificial sweetener, found in a myriad of dietetic or unsweetened products such as diet soda and Equal, occasionally triggers a migraine.

SULFITES. Sulfites are used to preserve some dried fruits, such as apricots. Sulfites are also often used in wine as a preservative. Many wine shops will be able to tell you which wines are sulfite-free.

12. Skipping Meals
Not only must you be careful of what you put in your mouth, but you need to be concerned if you put in nothing at all. If you find yourself frequently skipping meals, you may be inadvertently triggering a migraine. Even if you don't have hypoglycemia, when you don't eat, your blood sugar drops, which can be a migraine trigger. If you don't have time for a meal, at least try to eat a high-protein or complex-carbohydrate snack (not just something sugar-based) such as a hard-boiled egg. If your schedule is such that you cannot take a sit-down, away-from-the-office lunch break, either brown-bag your lunch or at least order some take-out food. Even fast food can be healthful if you're careful about what you select. (Baked potatoes and salads are widely available.)

13. Caffeine Withdrawal

Caffeine itself is generally not the culprit in triggering migraines, unless you drink truly excessive amounts, like two pots of coffee a day. What is more likely to be a trigger is an abrupt change in the level of your caffeine intake, as in caffeine withdrawal.

This can occur on weekends, on vacation, or when you're sick to your stomach. Caffeine withdrawal can occur when the amount of coffee (or soda) you drink during your leisure time fails to equal the amount you drink during your work-week. As with your sleep patterns, instead of making an abrupt change when the weekend rolls around, try to taper off on the amount you drink. For example, drink one less cup of coffee on Friday to prepare for the weekend, and don't go "cold turkey" on your cup of Joe when you head for the Caribbean. If you're feeling nauseated and the thought of coffee makes you more so, try drinking a Pepsi, Coke, or Mountain Dew. But remember that most colas contain about half the caffeine of an average cup of coffee.

If you wish to decrease or discontinue caffeine altogether, do so gradually. Decrease by one cola or one cup of coffee every day or two until you get to where you want to be. Bear in mind that the caffeine content of coffee varies, depending on how strong it is and how it's brewed. And a cup of tea usually contains a little less than half the caffeine of your average cup of coffee. Like coffee, teas vary. Black teas contain a caffeinelike substance, while green tea has very little caffeine. Most herbal teas contain none at all.

Don't forget that medications like Excedrin, Vivarin, and Fiorinal can also contain caffeine, usually in amounts greater than your average cup of coffee.

14. Alcohol

Alcohol is a very common trigger for migraine headaches, and not just when drunk to excess. Many migraineurs report that only half a glass of wine or a few sips of a cocktail can set off an attack.

Red wine is the form of alcohol most commonly listed as a migraine trigger. According to winemakers I've consulted in Oregon, which is known for its red wines, chemical analysis has revealed that there are more than three hundred different chemical compounds in many of the complex red wines. While some people may react to the sulfites used to preserve wines, others may react to one of the other compounds naturally occurring in red wine.

Red wine is not always to blame, however. I am able to drink most red wines but cannot enjoy Chardonnay or champagne without a migraine resulting. Other migraineurs have also reported a sensitivity to various white wines. So, as always, record what you drink in your migraine diary.

Some migraineurs register a sensitivity to beer, although this is not as common as that to wine. I have seen several patients who indicate a greater sensitivity to microbrews than to other beers.

Hard liquor is somewhat less likely to trigger a migraine than wine, but individual sensitivities do exist. Liqueurs tend to be more problematic than drier liquors like whiskey or vodka. I was recently persuaded to try a chocolate martini, which is made of vodka and Godiva chocolate liqueur. While it was very tasty, it did result in a headache for the two of us who tried it, both migraineurs. I suspect for me the trigger was the vodka, as I have never reacted to Godiva liqueur with a migraine before.

Some migraineurs report that their migraines are triggered by *any* type of alcohol.

SHOULD YOU GO ON A "MIGRAINE DIET"?

You may have heard about the so-called migraine diet, which is sometimes used to determine what your triggers are. It calls for going on a restrictive diet and then gradually adding one food item at a time and carefully charting your reactions to each food before adding another. This is a difficult and time-consuming process that many people are unable to follow. For that reason, along with the fact that only 25 percent of all migraineurs have food triggers, I only recommend it if you have frequent, difficult-to-control migraines.

For most migraineurs, keeping a migraine diary and being reasonably aware of what they eat or drink is adequate for determining migraine triggers.

Now that you've learned about some of the most common triggers and are scrupulously tracking your habits and patterns in a migraine diary, you are better able to identify what sets you off and what you can do to prevent the onset of a migraine. However, you may wonder why I've said almost nothing about what is perhaps the greatest of all major migraine triggers for women in their childbearing years—the onset of their menstrual period. That's because this phenomenon is so significant that I'm devoting an entire chapter to it. In my next chapter, I'll explain how and why your period can push you into having a migraine, and I'll tell you what you can do about it.

EATING OUT

Eating out at restaurants is one of the great pleasures of modern life, but if you're a migraineur, it can also be one of life's greatest perils. Once you've identified what—if any—your dietary migraine triggers are, the obvious course of action is to avoid them. But this is not possible if you don't know what's in the food you eat.

Most dining establishments will be only too glad to tell you how a dish is prepared, or if it contains onions, garlic, or cheese. Sometimes the dish can be prepared without the offending ingredient. If it can't, choose something else. However, let me warn you that restaurant personnel may not know whether there's MSG in the greens at the salad bar or in a house salad, as they often come pretreated and prepackaged. To play it safe, it's best to assume that the salad bar *does* contain MSG, unless the manager or someone else in the know is certain that it does not.

Many Chinese restaurants will serve food without MSG if you request it. But keep in mind that other ingredients in Chinese food, such as mushrooms or spices, can also act as migraine triggers.

ON THE FLY

Fast food and airport food are more difficult to contend with. These are sold by clerks who just heat them up and who have minimal (or no) connection with food preparation. Fast-food restaurants will supply you with nutritional information upon request. Airport food, however, comes from the supplier, and the people selling the food may not know the ingredients. When you're at McDonald's or an airport eatery, you might want to remember the information I've presented in the section on food triggers. Pay special attention to the fact that hot dogs contain nitrates/nitrites—a common trigger—as a preservative. And be wary of pizza, which can be a multitrigger food; it often contains preserved meats, olives, onions, garlic, and MSG.

Once you make a habit of exercising reasonable caution around restaurant food, most likely you, like most migraineurs, will be able to make eating out a pleasure.

CHAPTER
4

❖

The Menstrually Associated Migraine

BLAME IT ON YOUR HORMONES

The onset of menstruation is the single most significant trigger for women who suffer from migraine. About 60 percent of migraineurs in their childbearing years have headaches associated with their menstrual cycles. When you compare the migraine rates of children to those of adults, you'll see that female hormones figure prominently in the picture. Preadolescent girls and boys get migraines at about the same rate. But after puberty—during a woman's prime reproductive years, from ages fifteen to fifty—females outpace males in migraine incidence by a three-to-one ratio.

Hormonal changes are the chief reason women experience more migraines than men. Clearly, an estrogen connection exists. For many women with migraine, their first migraine occurred in relationship to some hormonal event—such as the onset of menses, the use of oral contraceptives, pregnancy, the postpartum period, or taking estrogen supplements as hormone replacement therapy during menopause. Ovulation is another significant hormonal trigger among women with migraine.

You might conclude, then, that hormones *cause* migraines. But this would be inaccurate. Hormones can trigger headaches in women who are genetically susceptible to migraine. However, not every woman reacts the same way to these commonplace triggers. (In some cases, estrogen replacement therapy and oral contraceptives can actually *prevent* migraines, while many women note relief from migraine headaches when pregnant.) Even among postmenopausal women, hormonal fluctuations continue to affect migraine.

NOT PMS

Let's straighten out one common fallacy right from the start: Menstrual migraine is *not* the same thing as premenstrual syndrome, PMS. PMS is a mood disorder occurring during a woman's premenstrual phase. It's often associated with fatigue, appetite change, nausea, breast swelling and tenderness, a bloated feeling, and backache. It does not necessarily involve headache. In fact, approximately half of women who suffer from PMS get headaches, but these are not necessarily migraines. A woman can have premenstrual migraine and not have PMS.

WHAT IS A MENSTRUAL MIGRAINE?

Experts in hormonal headache draw a distinction between premenstrual migraine and menstrual migraine. Premenstrual migraine begins from the seventh to the third day before a woman's period and gets better when the menstrual flow begins. Menstrual migraine is a headache that commences anytime from between one to two days before your period starts to when you begin bleeding and improves after the second or third day of menstruation. Occasionally menstrual migraines occur a day or two *after* a woman's period ends. However, one 1998 study showed that migraines were most likely to occur on the day before or on the first day of their menstrual period, with a "stable, linear decline" in headache probability thereafter.

Though some migraineurs have their only attacks just before or during their periods, many women who have migraines at other times of the month regularly experience them during menstruation as well. For this reason, I prefer the designation of "menstrually associated migraine" over "menstrual migraine." (For most laypeople and physicians, the two terms are virtually interchangeable.)

Menstrually associated migraine is migraine that occurs at the time of the menstrual period as well as at other times of the month. It is rarely associated with aura, but it can be. For many women, this is the most wrenchingly painful and difficult-to-treat headache of the month.

HOW IT FEELS

The pain that comes with the menstrually associated migraine is the same type of pain you feel with migraines at other times during your cycle, only it is far more intense. This migraine is often accompanied by the premenstrual symptoms of depression, back pain, pelvic fullness, and overall discomfort. And unfortunately, the menstrually associated migraine usually lasts longer than a nonmenstrual migraine, often two or three days. What's more, it shows greater resistance to the medications that usually work to combat nonmenstrual migraines—possibly because of alterations in receptors and a lower responsiveness to endorphins.

The good news is that migraine does not necessarily occur *every* month in affected women, although it does for some. I've noticed that among my patients who get menstrually associated migraine, roughly half contract these monster headaches every single menstrual cycle, while the other half get them more sporadically.

WHAT CAUSES MENSTRUALLY ASSOCIATED MIGRAINES?

The menstrually associated migraine is caused by the influence of a woman's hormonal interactions on someone who's genetically susceptible to migraine. To understand this, it's necessary to examine the hormonal fluctuations of normal menstrual cycles.

A complex interaction of hormones and neurotransmitters results in a woman's monthly cycle. The hypothalamus (which controls basic body functions) secretes gonadotropin-releasing hormone (GnRH), which stimulates the release of luteinizing hormone (LH) and follicle-stimulating hormone (FSH) from the pituitary gland.

FSH reaches a peak just before ovulation, stimulating an egg-containing follicle in the ovary to release the egg. FSH levels then drop, beginning to rise again premenstrually. By the time menstruation begins, FSH has risen to nearly the high levels of the preovulatory spike. This process prepares the next egg to be released by the ovary.

Luteinizing hormone levels peak sharply just before ovulation, ushering in the luteal phase. During ovulation, both FSH and LH stimulate the secretion of estrogen and progesterone by the ovaries. Estrogen levels rise before ovulation, fall just after, and increase somewhat again in the time between ovulation and menstruation. Estrogen drops sharply just before menstruation.

Progesterone levels are low during the preovulatory phase of your cycle. Progesterone begins to rise at ovulation and continues to rise during the luteal phase, falling sharply before menstruation.

For many years, it was unclear to doctors and researchers alike whether it was the progesterone fluctuation, the estrogen fluctuation, or some other hormonal pattern that might be responsible for menstrually associated migraines. Then, in a groundbreaking 1972 study, Australian neurologist B. W.

Somerville determined that menstrual migraines occurred *after* the fall of both estrogen and progesterone that occurs immediately before menstruation.

Somerville administered estrogen to study subjects who suffered from migraine during their premenstrual period to see what effect it might have on migraine occurrence. He found that giving estrogen premenstrually didn't prevent menstruation, but it delayed the migraine until estrogen levels fell. It has since been established that progesterone given premenstrually will delay menstruation but will not prevent migraine.

As a result of Somerville's work and related research, we now understand that menstrual migraine occurs directly after the time when estrogen is high and then drops. "Estrogen priming" is a period of sustained estrogen at high levels, whether occurring physiologically or by taking estrogen.

WHY ARE SOME IMMUNE TO MENSTRUAL MIGRAINE?

Since all menstruating migraineurs experience a similar spike in their estrogen levels each month, followed by a drop-off, why don't they all experience menstrual migraines? Why are 40 percent of women of childbearing age who have migraines apparently immune to menstrually associated migraines? The answers to these questions are not yet known, but they may well have to do with the genetics of migraine. It appears probable that more than one gene accounts for migraine susceptibility. This genetic variability could account for a subset of women with migraine who are not especially sensitive to hormonal fluctuations.

ESTROGEN'S EFFECT

Estrogen has many effects on the neurotransmitters in your brain. Both estrogen and progesterone enhance the brain's responsiveness to endorphins (naturally occurring opiatelike substances that block pain) and to opiate medications (such as codeine, hydrocodone, oxycodone, Demerol, morphine, and others).

Estrogen also increases the numbers of some types of brain receptors. Decreases in estrogen levels change the responsiveness of other receptors, rendering a woman more vulnerable to migraine. In addition, the monthly estrogen drop causes a decrease in platelet serotonin. Changes in serotonin balance are important in the genesis of a migraine.

The monthly drop in estrogen and progesterone also results in increased production of prostaglandins. Prostaglandins are circulating substances that cause uterine contractions, which result in menstrual cramps. Prostaglandins given to subjects experimentally brought about back pain that had been previously blocked by morphine. Intravenous infusion of one type of prostaglandin also resulted in nausea, flushing, diarrhea, cramping, a faint feeling, and difficulty concentrating. (Prostaglandins also have important beneficial functions, regulating smooth muscle contractions.)

Another answer to the origins of the menstrually associated migraine may lie in our circadian rhythm patterns. Many mammals do not have monthly cycles but do have seasonal breeding patterns. This seasonal breeding is triggered by melatonin, a hormone secreted in various levels during the day in relation to cycles of lightness and dark. This hormone, in turn, triggers the release of GnRH. As in humans, GnRH release triggers LH and FSH, preparing the ovaries for hormone secretion and ultimately for conception.

In humans, the relationship between melatonin and the reproductive cycle is less clear. Some headache experts theorize that there is altered melatonin metabolism associated with menstrual migraine (though we still don't know if it's a result of more, less, or an uneven production of melatonin). We do know that affected women lack the fluctuation in melatonin excretion experienced by nonaffected women. What's more, a Finnish study demonstrated that variations in day length occurring in high northern latitudes affect the conception rate. So it might be reasonable to postulate that melatonin could affect reproductive cycles as well as related migraines.

There are several studies that link possible alterations in the brain's magnesium levels to the menstrually associated migraine. At present, however, it's not been established whether these alterations would enhance your susceptibility to menstrually associated migraines. However, until further studies are conducted using strict controls, the mechanism of migraine triggered by hormonal events remains uncertain. As research into this area continues, the future should deliver some promising answers.

MANAGING YOUR MENSTRUALLY ASSOCIATED MIGRAINES

In many cases of menstrually associated migraine, the headache is treated when it occurs, and prevention is not required. For many women, the medications that combat their usual migraines also work effectively for their menstrually associated migraines.

The "first line" of treatment for menstrually associated migraines consists of acute migraine medications such as nonsteroidal anti-inflammatories naproxen sodium (Aleve or Anaprox); ketoprofen (Orudis KT or Actron); flurbiprofen (Ansaid) and others; ergotamine (Cafergot, Ergomar, or Wigraine); or dihydroergotamine (DHE-45 or Migranal), and medications like sumatriptan (Imitrex), zolmitriptan (Zomig), or rizatriptan (Maxalt). Research has shown that sumatriptan (Imitrex) reduces the moderate or severe menstrually associated migraine to a mild headache or no headache in 70 to 80 percent of occurrences. (Read more about medications in Chapter 7.)

MINIPREVENTION

Unfortunately, some women find that their menstrually associated migraines are especially resistant to treatment and their usual medication is not as effective as it is for their non-menstrual migraines. When acute treatment doesn't work, I recommend that migraineurs try intermittent "miniprevention." This works best among women who can accurately predict when their periods will occur. Various regimens of intermittent prevention are available. They can consist of taking an anti-inflammatory medication for three to seven days premenstrually or taking ergot medications or a triptan medication like sumatriptan (Imitrex) for a few days premenstrually.

Diana, a patient of mine, was usually able to banish her nonmenstrual migraines with naproxen sodium (Aleve) or iso-metheptene mucate, dichloralphenazone, or acetaminophen (Midrin, Duradrin, or Midchlor). However, these medications barely put a dent in her menstrually associated migraines. Fortunately, Diana's menstrually associated migraines have responded to sumatriptan (Imitrex). And at least one study confirmed these results. It showed promising outcomes among women who took a regimen of 25 milligrams of sumatriptan (Imitrex) three times a day starting two or three days prior to the expected day of headache onset. Headaches did not occur *at all* in over 52 percent of the women participating in the study, and headache severity was cut by half or more among 42 percent.

Prior to beginning on a migraine-miniprevention program with amitriptyline (Elavil), another patient, Pam, had two or three migraines every month, one of which was menstrually associated. Once I started Pam on amitriptyline, her migraine incidence was reduced to one severe headache a day or two before her period started. However, after increasing her amitriptyline dose and having her take it daily, Pam has been fortunate enough to reduce that number to just two or three mild migraines—both nonmenstrual and menstrual—per year!

Occasionally, miniprevention consists of the usual migraine-prevention medications (tricyclic antidepressants, beta blockers, calcium channel blockers, or anticonvulsant medications) given for ten to fourteen days premenstrually. This form of treatment is useful for women who experience only menstrual migraines. It also helps women whose non-menstrual migraines are manageable with acute treatment and who do not need preventative medications throughout the entire month.

Women who do need daily preventative medications may find all but their menstrual migraine effectively suppressed each month. Increasing the dose of their usual preventative medication premenstrually may help.

Another strategy sometimes used to treat menstrually associated migraine is the premenstrual use of estrogen supplementation. A low-dose estrogen skin patch used three to seven days premenstrually can often prevent or diminish a menstrual migraine attack.

MANAGING YOUR MIGRAINES IF YOU'RE TAKING BIRTH CONTROL PILLS

For women who are on oral contraceptives, a change in the form of pill they take can help by extending the number of days they take estrogen. Most oral contraceptives provide twenty-one days of hormone-containing pills and seven days of blanks. Newer oral contraceptives have been developed that reduce the estrogen dose and extend its use for all but two days in the cycle. This limits the extent of the estrogen decrease premenstrually.

Another way to control menstrual migraines by using oral contraceptives is to take the Pill continuously for three to five months. This still results in a period of "estrogen priming," followed by estrogen withdrawal. This will give you a menstrual period and, most likely, a migraine, too, but at least you can plan for it, and it only occurs every few months.

Allowing menstruation every three to five months diminishes the risk of uterine cancer that would be associated with continuous estrogen use.

OTHER TREATMENT STRATEGIES

For women with difficult-to-treat menstrually associated migraine, other strategies are necessary. These involve the suppression of various sorts of female hormones.

Bromocriptine Treatment

In a study published in a 1997 issue of *Neurology*, twenty-four women with menstrual migraines who were unresponsive to the standard treatments were given continuous bromocriptine (Parlodel). Seventy five percent of the subjects experienced at least 25 percent fewer attacks. Bromocriptine has also been used intermittently. However, not everyone tolerates this medication; nausea is its most common side effect.

I have had several patients who could not tolerate the medication. Charlene, however, had been on the Pill for no other reason than to ensure that her menstrually associated migraines occurred on weekends, as she lost three or four days each month to menstrual migraine. Since beginning on bromocriptine, she has reduced this to one or two mild headache days monthly.

Antiestrogen Medications

Antiestrogen medications have also been proposed to treat menstrually associated migraines. Danazol (Danocrine), a male hormone medication, has been used for this purpose. However, I do not frequently prescribe it. Because it is a masculinizing medication, many women dislike its adverse effects, which include the coarsening of body hair and sometimes facial-hair development. With prolonged usage, a deepening of the voice and even decreased breast size can occur. To limit these masculinizing effects, danazol is sometimes given only premenstrually and during menses.

Tamoxifen (Nolvadex), a medication usually used to treat breast cancer, is another antiestrogen medication that has been suggested for menstrual migraines. In a 1990 article in *Neurology*, a single case was reported of a woman using tamoxifen for PMS who noted improvement of her menstrually associated migraines. A noted expert on hormonally related migraine, Stephen D. Silberstein, M.D., who's based at Thomas Jefferson University Headache Center in Philadelphia, has recommended using tamoxifen for seven days prior to onset of the menstrual period.

For severe, seemingly intractable cases of menstrually associated migraine, leuprolide acetate (Lupron)—a drug that induces chemical menopause—may help. This medication does not have the masculinizing effects of danazol. However, not all migraineurs are comfortable with such a radical strategy.

In a 1995 issue of *Headache Quarterly*, researchers reported on their use of leuprolide acetate in a study of twenty-nine women with menstrual migraines that lasted more than one day each month and had hitherto resisted treatment. Each woman described her headaches as "incapacitating" and "nonresponsive" to ergotamine with caffeine and codeine. So severe were their migraines that each had required emergency-room care four or more times in the preceding year. Over two years, fourteen of the women studied experienced a decrease in headache severity by 50 percent or more when using leuprolide. Five others showed a lesser benefit. The remaining subjects either dropped out of the study because of side effects or experienced a significant worsening of their migraines. (Because leuprolide suppresses estrogen production of the ovary, the women who continued treatment were given "add-back" estrogen supplementation to counteract the effects of chemical menopause.)

Bromocriptine, danazol, and leuprolide acetate should only be used in carefully selected women because all three medications have significant side effects. Women with menstrually associated migraines should try the other treatment strategies described above before resorting to these medications.

IS TOTAL HYSTERECTOMY THE ANSWER?

In the past, hysterectomy with removal of the ovaries (oophorectomy) has been used by some physicians to treat severe menstrually associated migraines. Less than half the women who have taken this route have experienced improvement. In most cases the headaches no longer occur predictably each month.

A patient named Helen who suffered from severe menstrual migraines each month when she was in her thirties was able to gain some measure of relief by taking aspirin, butalbital, and caffeine (Fiorinal) with codeine. At age thirty-seven she opted for a hysterectomy, hoping to free herself of migraines once and for all. Unfortunately, it didn't work out that way. Now approaching fifty, Helen still gets migraines, but today she manages her pain with the preventative medication verapamil (Calan, Isoptin, or Verelan) and the occasional injection of sumatriptan (Imitrex).

A complete hysterectomy performed solely to relieve migraines is not currently recommended.

Other hormonally induced headaches that are similar to naturally occurring menstrually associated migraines are headaches that occur during the pill-free interval in women on oral contraceptives. This, too, is a headache precipitated by a period of estrogen priming (the active pill phase), followed by estrogen withdrawal, when you either take nothing or take blanks, usually sugar pills. This type of headache usually goes away once the active estrogen-containing pill is resumed.

Migraines may become worse when a woman begins taking oral contraceptives. Studies report an increase in frequency and severity of migraine attacks in 18 to 50 percent of cases. Yet up to 35 percent of women noted improvement in migraines once they started taking the Pill. And, in several studies, no difference was found in headache frequency, regardless of whether a woman was given the Pill or a placebo.

This variability in response may reflect the many doses and formulations of various oral contraceptives; they don't all contain the same ingredients or the same amounts of ingredients. Occasionally, a woman experiences migraines for the first time after starting oral contraceptives.

A 1975 study conducted by Lee Kudrow, M.D., of the California Medical Clinic for Headache in Encino, reported that of women who had not experienced migraines before and began having them when starting oral contraceptives, only 40 percent had a family history of migraine. Among women on birth control pills who had migraines before starting the Pill, 72 percent had a family history of migraine. This study pointed to the probable role of estrogen as the precipitating factor in oral contraceptive–induced migraine. The lower rate of family history of migraine suggests that many of these women would not have developed migraine had they not been exposed to the estrogen in oral contraceptives.

Treatment of migraine in women on oral contraceptives does not differ from treatment of migraine in general. The Pill is compatible with migraine medications. If a migraineur on the Pill develops daily headaches, a migraine aura for the first time, or a sudden severe headache, she should contact her doctor for a neurologic evaluation. In this case, oral contraceptives may need to be discontinued. But these instances are rare indeed.

Women with migraines have a slightly increased risk of stroke compared with the general female population. And the use of oral contraceptives can notch up that risk even more. (However, the lower the dose of estrogen in the birth control pills, the lower the increase of stroke risk.) Female migraineurs on the Pill should not smoke because smoking further increases stroke risk.

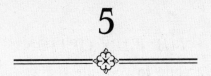

Migraine and Pregnancy

For every expectant mother, pregnancy is a time of joy and fear, of great expectations and nagging anxieties. But if you suffer from migraines, pregnancy—or the prospect of having a baby—will introduce an added set of concerns. Doubtless you'll worry about how your migraines will affect your pregnancy and how your pregnancy will affect your migraines. Your mind may begin swimming with a number of troubling possibilities, such as:

- Will my migraines persist, worsen, or disappear over the course of the pregnancy?
- If I have to take medications for migraines, could they harm the fetus?
- Am I really up to the job of night feedings, diaperings, and taking care of a sick baby when I come down with a debilitating migraine attack and am barely able to function myself?
- Once the baby is born, will I be able to breast-feed?

In this chapter, I'll tackle these and other questions and summarize the research findings that will give you insight into the experience of your fellow migraineurs during pregnancy.

THE BABY OPTION

While adding a child to your life is always a momentous decision, when you suffer from migraine, the question of time and pain management takes on an added dimension. If you're thinking about becoming pregnant, you'll want to know the facts so you can make an informed decision. What I recommend to my patients who are considering the baby option is to base their decision on their own personal, emotional, and financial situation. As with any prospective mother, you'll want to take your health picture into account, which in your case includes your history of migraine.

There are dozens of excellent self-help books on the market that can guide you in making a sound decision on whether to get pregnant and how to prepare for an optimal pregnancy. In my view, the question of whether or not to become a parent is such a large one—a life question—that unless your migraines are debilitating to the extreme, they should not be the deciding factor in ruling out pregnancy. That is not to say that I think every woman should become a parent. But if having a child has always been in your dreams and in your life plan, you might be selling yourself short to summarily rule it out because of your migraines and associated fears.

IF YOU DECIDE TO GO FOR IT

If you decide to become pregnant, it's a good idea to alert your OB/GYN and your primary physician about your migraines ahead of time, so that you can discuss what strategy to pursue should you continue to suffer from headaches during pregnancy. It is better to make a plan that you may never use than to wait until you're in the throes of an agonizing migraine to frantically try to reach your physician for a last-minute prescription. When making your plan, you may want to consider pursuing some of the alternative/nonpharmaceutical therapies, which will not harm your fetus. (Read about these techniques in depth in Chapter 8.)

Bear in mind that just because you make a pain-management plan doesn't mean you have to follow it if your circumstances change. Once you're actually pregnant, real experience will reveal if and how your headache pattern will change. Then you and your physician can make medication and treatment decisions based on your needs of the moment, taking into consideration your primary desire to protect the health of your baby, along with your own comfort and well-being.

THE GOOD NEWS ABOUT PREGNANCY

The good news about pregnancy is that it cuts most migraineurs a lucky break. Most women will see their migraines improve or disappear altogether during pregnancy. In fact, sometimes the state of pregnancy is so pain-free and euphoric for migraineurs that they half-regret delivering the baby. Marianna, a thirty-one-year-old client, joked with me after having her first baby that her headaches had improved so much during the course of her pregnancy—and that her pregnancy had been so trouble-free—that if she could swing it, she'd remain pregnant continuously. (In fact, after Marianna's first baby, a strapping girl, was born, she went on to two more "dream" pregnancies.)

However, some women are not so lucky and will experience a worsening of their migraines during pregnancy. And a few will begin having migraines for the first time while pregnant. The problem is you won't really know if you'll be among the lucky majority or the accursed few until after you've become pregnant.

WHAT ARE THE ODDS?

Medical research shows that the menstrual migraineur has a better chance of improvement during pregnancy than the nonmenstrual migraineur. During pregnancy, both estrogen and progesterone rise steadily higher until delivery. As demonstrated in Chapter 4, high estrogen levels protect women from hormonally sensitive headaches. It would stand to reason, then, that menstrual migraine sufferers should improve or become headache-free when pregnant, and that the greatest improvement would be expected in the third trimester, when estrogen levels are at their peak. For the majority of women with migraine who become pregnant, Mother Nature deals a lucky break.

A review of the medical research about migraine and pregnancy confirms these findings. If you're like the women studied, your prospects for a positive pregnancy experience are great. A landmark 1966 study of 252 pregnant women with a history of migraines prior to becoming pregnant showed that nearly two-thirds, or 64 percent, of the women with menstrually associated migraines improved during the course of their pregnancies. However, only about half, or 48 percent, of the women with nonmenstrual migraines showed improvement. A 1990 study delivered even more encouraging results, showing that 86 percent of menstrual migraineurs improved with pregnancy, compared with only 52 percent of women with nonmenstrual migraine. One study found that women whose migraines began when their periods did were the most likely to see headache improvements when pregnant.

As a result of these and other studies, most women are told by their physicians that they can expect their migraines to go away when they're pregnant or at least to improve in the third trimester. All of these studies, however, were conducted by surveying women about their headaches *after* they had delivered. Why is this significant?

Dawn Marcus, M.D., and associates studied forty-nine pregnant women with chronic headaches, eighteen of whom had migraine. They began their monitoring in the first trimester. The women recorded data regarding their headaches, or lack thereof, four times each day throughout pregnancy. For most, there was little change in headache occurrence in pregnancy compared to prepregnant levels, and no improvement in the third trimester over early pregnancy. When the same women were surveyed after delivery, however, it was their perception that they had experienced continued improvement during pregnancy, with a recurrence of headache in the postpartum period. It may have been that they felt better overall, despite continuing to experience migraines. Or it may simply be that we don't remember pain very well.

So while I can't promise you that you won't have migraines while pregnant, it is likely that you'll feel better in the third trimester. And it is likely that you'll look back on this stage of pregnancy with positive memories.

TREATING MIGRAINES WHEN YOU'RE PREGNANT

If you begin or continue to experience migraines when pregnant, what can you do about it? Must you suffer with no medication for nine long months? Or can you take the drugs that helped you through before you were expecting?

NONMEDICATION PAIN MANAGEMENT

As the first line of defense and the least risky way to prevent and handle your migraines while pregnant, I recommend that my patients follow nonmedication strategies. These include physical therapy, biofeedback, massage therapy, acupuncture, and relaxation (more on these in Chapter 8). If you've never before considered such alternative treatments to manage pain, your incentive is great at this time to investigate one or more of the following:

- *physical therapy:* a directed program incorporating massage, joint mobilization, and strengthening exercises directed at specific muscle groups for the relief of pain and spasm;
- *biofeedback:* a technique that many migraineurs find useful through which you learn to relax muscles using

a machine that shows you a picture of your muscle tension;

- *massage:* a familiar, pleasurable, hands-on-your-body rub-down that stimulates circulation and relaxes the muscles;
- *relaxation therapy:* self-guided techniques to bring about overall mind-body relaxation;
- *acupuncture:* the Chinese practice of inserting needles into various points in your body to stimulate the production of endorphins to relieve pain.

If you are skeptical of alternative medicine and have tended to dismiss it as being out of the mainstream, consider one major study. Lisa Scharff, M.D., and her colleagues at the University of Pittsburgh Pain Evaluation and Treatment Institute studied thirty pregnant women with headaches who were treated with either biofeedback, relaxation training, or physical therapy. These forms of treatment benefited a whopping 80 percent of the women studied, who reported significant relief in their headache diaries. These same women were followed after delivery. Fully 67 percent of the women who'd received these alternative treatments still had a significant decrease in their headaches for up to one year after giving birth.

Another nonmedication option: If you can get the go-ahead from your physician, you might try magnesium supplementation for migraine prevention. Several studies have shown benefit for some migraineurs. Magnesium sulfate is also used to treat eclampsia, a complication of pregnancy that causes high blood pressure and kidney abnormalities and can cause seizures and other brain abnormalities. Magnesium supplements are probably safe in pregnancy, although we do not yet know the optimal dose for migraine prevention.

CATEGORIES OF MEDICATIONS AND PREGNANCY RISKS

As effective as they are in promoting overall good health in most people, including many women with migraine, alternative techniques are simply not successful for all migraineurs, nor for all headaches in a given woman. If you do resort to medications to control pain during pregnancy, take heart, you're not alone. Demographic studies have shown that about two-thirds of all pregnant women take some sort of medication at some time during their pregnancy. And fully 50 percent of all pregnant women take a medication in their first trimester, which is the most critical time for the normal development of the fetus.

Still, when you do take a medication, you must ask yourself: What effect could this have on my baby? While only about twenty drugs have been proven to cause birth defects, many medications—in fact, most—have not yet been tested. Other medications may not cause severe problems but may delay fetal growth and cause minor damage to internal organs, minor birth defects, or behavioral changes in the child after birth. Major birth defects are those that require surgical correction—such as esophageal atresia (an esophagus that ends in a blind pouch and requires surgical correction) and those that result in miscarriage or stillbirth. Minor defects are physical or cosmetic imperfections such as birthmarks, skin tags, and the like.

ANALYZING THE CAUSES OF BIRTH DEFECTS

Fortunately, having migraine headaches alone does not harm the developing fetus or attach any sort of enhanced risk of negative outcomes to a pregnancy. And you can take comfort in knowing that there is no increased rate of miscarriages or stillbirths among migraineur mothers or any higher percentage of birth defects among the offspring of mothers with migraines. What's more, there are no specific birth defects linked to mothers with migraines. Only if a woman suffers a prolonged migraine with vomiting leading to dehydration is there any risk to the baby she carries.

Turning to medications without first considering the impact they might have on your unborn child can put your baby at increased risk for birth defects (this, of course, is also true for nonmigraineur pregnant women who take medication). The chart that follows shows which common medications are considered best and worst. You do need to be extremely careful when you're pregnant about what medications you put into your system. Major birth defects occur in 2 to 3 percent of all pregnancies in the general population, while minor birth defects occur in 7 to 10 percent of all live births. About 25 percent of all birth defects in the general population are genetically related, and about 23 percent are thought to be due to drug or alcohol exposure. A probable cause cannot be identified in the other 52 percent of cases.

MEDICATIONS AND THEIR PREGNANCY RISKS

If you suspect you'll need to take medication to alleviate your pain during pregnancy, you might want to study the

HOW DO WE LEARN ABOUT SIDE EFFECTS OF DRUGS?

Knowledge about the possible effects of many medications on the developing fetus is usually quite limited. This is because in 1977 the FDA prohibited the testing of new drugs on pregnant women. Now the only way to garner information is by studying women who take medications before they realize they're pregnant or those who must take medications for serious and potentially life-threatening conditions, such as serious infection and high blood pressure.

If you have taken either sumatriptan (Imitrex or Imigran) or naratriptan (Amerge or Naramig) before you realized you were pregnant and would like to help further research, have your doctor or nurse-midwife sign you up for a voluntary pregnancy registry established by the drug manufacturer Glaxo Wellcome by calling 1 (888) 825-5249, ext. 39441. Thus far, no evidence exists that either medication results in birth defects above the baseline rate, but more data is needed.

following information in advance so that you'll know what is safe to use and what you'll want to avoid. Because of its concern over the possible impact of medications on a developing fetus, the Food and Drug Administration (FDA) has assigned five classes of risk for medications in pregnancy. They are:

- Class A: No risk in controlled studies
- Class B: No evidence of risk; no controlled studies exist
- Class C: Risk to humans has not been ruled out
- Class D: Positive evidence of probable risk to humans in human or animal studies
- Class X: Not recommended during pregnancy

Medications commonly used for acute treatment of migraine are classified as follows:

MEDICATION	Class
MINOR ANALGESICS	
aspirin	C
acetaminophen (Tylenol)	B
caffeine	B
ibuprofen (Motrin)	B
naproxen (Naprosyn)	B
indomethacin (Indocin)	B
ketoprofen (Orudis KT)	B
NARCOTICS	
butorphanol (Stadol)	C
codeine	C
meperidine (Demerol)	B
methadone	B
morphine	B
propoxyphene (Darvocet)	C
STEROIDS	
dexamethasone (Decadron)	C
prednisone (Meticorten)	B

MEDICATION	Class
ERGOT DERIVATIVES	
ergotamine tartrate (Ergomar, Ergostat)	X
dihydroergotamine (DHE-45, Migranal)	X
TRIPTANS	
sumatriptan	
(Imitrex, Imigran)	C
naratriptan (Amerge)	C
zolmitriptan (Zomig)	C
rizatriptan (Maxalt)	C
MISCELLANEOUS	
butalbital (in Fiorinal, Fioricet, Esgic, others)	C
phenobarbital (—)	D
diazepam (Valium)	D
clonazepam (Klonopin)	D

ANTINAUSEA MEDICATIONS

	Class
ANTIHISTAMINE TYPE	
cyproheptadine (Periactin)	B
meclizine (Antivert)	B
(Dramamine)	B
(Marezine)	B
NEUROLEPTIC TYPE	
chlorpromazine (Thorazine)	C
prochlorperazine (Compazine)	C
haloperidol (Haldol)	C
metoclopramide (Reglan)	B
MISCELLANEOUS	
(Emetrol)	B
Vitamin B-6	B

Preventative medications for migraine fall into the following classes of risk:

MEDICATION	Class
BETA BLOCKERS	
metoprolol (Lopressor)	B
propanolol (Inderal)	C
nadolol (Corgard)	C
timolol (Blocadren)	C
atenolol (Tenormin)	C
TRICYCLIC ANTIDEPRESSANTS	
amitriptyline (Elavil)	D
nortriptyline (Pamelor)	D
doxepin (Sinequan)	C
protriptyline (Vivactil)	C
SSRI ANTIDEPRESSANTS	
fluoxetine (Prozac)	B
sertraline (Zoloft)	B
paroxetine (Paxil)	C
venlafaxine (Effexor)	C
nefazodone (Serzone)	C
CALCIUM CHANNEL BLOCKERS	
verapamil (Calan, Verelan, Isoptin)	C
nifedipine (Procardia)	C
diltiazem (Dilacor)	C
MISCELLANEOUS	
divalproex (Depakote)	D
methysergide (Sansert)	D
gabapentin (Neurontin)	C

When you are hit by a migraine, my best recommendation is to treat each headache as it occurs. Only in extreme cases do I prescribe preventative medications during pregnancy. When they are absolutely necessary, I always recommend the safest possible medications at the lowest effective dose.

Beta blockers are frequently prescribed for women with high blood pressure during pregnancy and can also be used for migraine prevention. They are occasionally associated with growth delay in the fetus. Amitriptyline (Elavil) has been used in the past for serious depression; it is still occasionally used for migraine suppression. It must be discontinued at least two weeks before the due date to avoid infant sedation, respiratory distress, or feeding difficulties.

Nonsteroidal anti-inflammatory medications are felt to be generally safe in the first and second trimesters of pregnancy. Ketoprofen (Orudis KT or Actron), ibuprofen (Motrin), flurbiprofen (Ansaid), and naproxen (Naprosyn) have been listed as probably the most likely to be helpful in the relief of your migraine pain yet fairly safe for your baby's development. Warning: Anti-inflammatory medications *cannot* be used in the third trimester because they increase the risks of pulmonary problems in the infant and the risks of prolonged or delayed labor, toxemia, or hemorrhage in the mother.

CAUSE FOR CONCERN

If your migraines worsen during pregnancy—or you get them for the first time—your doctor may be concerned that it could be something other than migraine. While most likely this is not the case, it is a valid concern. Some conditions that can mimic migraine occur more frequently in pregnancy than otherwise, among them stroke, subarachnoid hemorrhage, thrombosis (or blood clot) forming in cerebral veins, or pituitary tumor (usually not cancer).

Some complications of pregnancy can cause headaches that may resemble migraines. These include gestational hypertension (high blood pressure related to pregnancy), toxemia, and choriocarcinoma (an extremely rare and unfortunate condition in which the placenta itself becomes cancerous).

Diagnostic testing during pregnancy is never ideal. Obviously, physicians don't want to order any unnecessary X rays in pregnant women; however, the risk of a head CT scan is much, much lower than the risk of bleeding into your brain, or clotting and having a stroke. If your symptoms strongly indicate one of these conditions, testing may be necessary. Such tests are safest if they can wait until you're in the third trimester of pregnancy (though this may not always be possible).

Other nonmigraine conditions causing headache occur at the same rates whether or not you are pregnant: sinusitis, meningitis, vasculitis (inflammation of blood vessels), or brain tumors. (See Chapters 1 and 2 for a discussion of headaches other than migraines.)

THE POSTPARTUM MIGRAINE

About 39 percent of all pregnant women report a migraine-like headache in the first week postpartum, most commonly on the third to sixth day after delivering their child. And 58 percent of migraineurs who give birth will develop a postpartum headache. It is generally milder than their usual migraine attacks and tends to last longer.

In a small percentage of women, headache occurs for the first time in the postpartum period. A 1993 study reported that 4.5 percent of the women studied developed migraines for the first time during the postpartum period.

Another study revealed that 3.6 percent of all women followed had headaches postpartum (up to three months after delivery), and 1.4 percent of these headaches met the criteria for migraines.

WHAT CAUSES POSTPARTUM MIGRAINES?

Estrogen reaches very high levels by the end of the third trimester. After delivery, estrogen levels drop precipitously.

This is essentially a period of estrogen priming followed by an abrupt drop in estrogen, similar to the smaller estrogen rise and fall that causes menstrual migraines. It is not surprising, therefore, that this hormonal shift can bring on a migraine in those susceptible to it.

The postpartum migraine can be treated as any other migraine would be with whatever medication you've found helpful before you got pregnant—unless you wish to breast-feed. Then the baby's health must be taken into consideration.

BREAST FEEDING AND MIGRAINE

In deciding how to treat migraines in the breast-feeding woman, physicians need to consider whether or not the medication in question is secreted into breast milk and, if so, whether in significant quantities that might affect the baby. The American Academy of Pediatrics Committee on Drugs has classified medications for breast-feeding mothers as follows:

- usually compatible
- use with caution
- effects unknown but of concern
- requires temporary cessation of breast feeding
- contraindicated, or not recommended

Medications that are often used to treat headaches classified as "usually compatible" include acetaminophen (Tylenol), caffeine, nonsteroidal anti-inflammatories (Ansaid, Aleve, Advil), narcotic analgesics, prochlorperazine (Compazine), beta blockers (Atenolol or Propanolol), adrenergic blockers (clonidine), calcium channel blockers (Verapamil), carbamazepine (Tegretol), divalproex (Depakote), and steroids (prednisone). Some experts feel the safest nonsteroidal anti-inflammatory medications to use while breast feeding are ibuprofen (Advil, Motrin), flurbiprofen (Ansaid), diclofenac (Voltaren or Cataflam), and mefanamic acid (Ponstel).

Medications are classified into "use-with-caution" category for breast-feeding women for reasons ranging from infant sedation to the potential for prolonged bleeding. These include aspirin, barbiturates, methysergide (Sansert), sumatriptan (Imitrex, Imigran), and SSRI antidepressants—fluoxetine (Prozac), sertraline (Zoloft), paroxetine (Paxil), and venlafaxine (Effexor).

Medications in the "effects-unknown-but-of-concern" category are metoclopramide (Reglan), chlorpromazine (Thorazine), benzodiazepine drugs (Valium, Xanax, Ativan, Klonopin, and others), and tricyclic antidepressants—amitriptyline (Elavil), nortriptyline (Pamelor), doxepin (Sinequan), protriptyline (Vivactil), imipramine (Tofranil), and desipramine (Norpramin).

Some medications commonly used to treat migraine—cyproheptadine (Periactin), ergotamines (Cafergot, Ergomar, Wigraine), and dihydroergotamine (DHE-45, Migranal)—should not be used by breast-feeding women. (Make sure any doctor you work with knows you are breast-feeding your baby.)

TAKING MEDICATION *AFTER* FEEDING MAY HELP

One way to minimize risk to your baby from headache medications is to wait to take a medication until a feeding is over. Most medications for the acute treatment of migraine act fairly rapidly, which means the peak blood (and milk) levels occur within one to three hours of ingestion. If your baby goes that long between feedings, most of the medication will be out of your system by the next time you feed your baby. If your baby does feed sooner, pump and discard breast milk and feed the baby breast milk you have previously pumped and set aside in the refrigerator.

THE BREAST FEEDING HEADACHE

The "lactational cephalgia," a fancy name for a headache associated with breast feeding, is rare. Some experts believe that this headache, which occurs as the baby is put to the breast, can be attributed to a hormone called oxytocin. Oxytocin is released when the "let-down reflex" occurs (when milk leaves the ducts in the breast tissue, filling the space beneath the nipple, and flows out).

Once you have weaned the baby, you may resume your usual medication treatment for migraines. If you anticipate breast-feeding your child for a year or more, you may wish to explore nonmedication strategies for headache control.

NO GUILT TRIPS, PLEASE

If your postpartum migraine pain is severe and you simply must have medications that worked for you before pregnancy, don't feel guilty if you must resort to feeding your baby infant formula. Your baby will doubtless be a whole lot happier with a calm and present mother who's giving him a bottle than with a mother who's frazzled, medication-deprived, and at wit's end. This is true especially after the baby is three months old.

If you approach your pregnancy and postpregnancy period with a sound game plan, having a baby should bring you the wonder and exhilaration that all mothers feel—along with the usual discomforts of pregnancy and agonies of childbirth itself. There's a good chance that pregnancy will give you a respite from your migraines. But I always counsel my clients to plan strategies in advance of getting pregnant for confronting migraine pain. Once you put your proverbial ducks in a row, you should be able proceed with your pregnancy plans without undue worry. Then, when your bundle of joy does arrive on the scene, you'll be in good shape to handle her feeding as well as every aspect of her care.

CHAPTER

6

━━━◆━━━

Migraine and Menopause

Since migraines are so closely linked to menstrual periods in many women, you would think that with the onset of menopause you'd be home free, that your migraines would be a thing of the past.

Unfortunately, it doesn't always work out that way. Sad to say, some women actually experience a worsening of migraines in their menopausal years due to the hormonal fluctuations associated with the "change of life." In some cases, women are revisited by migraines they thought were a distant—if painful—memory.

Victoria, fifty-two, is a case in point. She had suffered from migraines throughout her twenties, having contracted her first at age nineteen and her last after she married at age thirty. But about three years ago, with menopause coming on, her migraines returned with a vengeance. "The onset for me is typically at three in the morning," she said. "I wake up and the pain is one-sided, sometimes left and sometimes right. It's a hard, constant pain, incapacitating at times." Victoria's menopausal migraines are different in character from the ones she experienced during her salad days. They're more frequent but less sensitive to sound and noise, and rarely do they induce nausea. "When I was younger, I was so sick, I'd have to go into a dark room and stay there. Now, with the help of Imitrex in nasal-spray form, I can work through my headaches."

You may get lucky and see your migraines disappear as you enter menopause. Or you may find that with menopause your migraines will persist or worsen, or even return after a hiatus, like Victoria's did. Let's look at some solutions that can help you manage—and even "work through"—your menopausal migraines.

Migraineurs, of course, differ considerably, and one solution will not necessarily suit all. What's more, when tackling the menopausal migraine, it's also necessary to take into account the many ways in which various treatments for menopause can impact migraine.

PERIMENOPAUSE AND MENOPAUSE

Perimenopause refers to a period of several years in which your hormones are declining but you have not completely ceased menstruation and your ovaries have not yet stopped functioning altogether. During perimenopause, your menstrual periods may change in character and duration, and they may occur infrequently. Menopause commences when your menstrual periods have ceased for more than one year; most commonly, this happens when a woman is in her mid- to late forties or older.

Although the parents of a twelve-year-old girl may feel as if their little daughter has been transformed into an adolescent overnight, in fact the process has taken place over the course of several years. Likewise, the changes that occur in a woman's body as she approaches menopause are gradual. And unless it happens as the result of the surgical removal of her ovaries, menopause isn't triggered by some internal on/ off switch. In perimenopause you may begin to notice a number of changes that come on over time. You may find your sex drive to be less robust than previously. Vaginal dryness, which can make intercourse painful, is often a problem. Your menstrual flow may become lighter or heavier, and your periods are likely to become less predictable. You may experience night sweats—in which you wake up feeling suddenly and inexplicably hot and in some cases have thoroughly soaked the sheets. Night sweats (not the same thing as hot flashes, which women describe as feeling like they're burning up inside) may precede menopause by as much as ten years. Some women report emotional symptoms, such as irritability, lack of concentration, oversentimentality, sensitivity, and mood swings.

These symptoms are all part of the natural process that your body is undergoing as it prepares to make fundamental change. As discussed in Chapter 4, studies demonstrate that a period of estrogen priming followed by withdrawal of estrogen occurs monthly, to coincide with a woman's cycle of ovulation and menstrual flow. Among genetically susceptible women, this cycle results in menstrual migraines. In a way, you can consider all your reproductive years as a period of estrogen priming, with menopause as a gradual withdrawal. Thus, women who are genetically susceptible develop more migraines perimenopausally than they did previously.

HORMONE REPLACEMENT THERAPY

About 75 percent of all women in English-speaking countries make the transition into menopause without significant problems and without the need for medical assistance. If these women do have annoying symptoms, such as hot flashes and emotionally charged spells, they usually end within two years, without treatment.

The treatment of menopause through hormone replacement therapy (HRT) remains controversial. Some women believe that HRT "medicalizes" a naturally occurring state, and that menopausal women should not be considered sick or deficient. However, there's no debating the fact that they *are* deficient in estrogen, and this deficiency carries health consequences. As we analyze the menopausal migraine, you'll find that this state of estrogen deficiency plays a central role in both the cause and management of your migraines.

ALTERNATING HORMONE REGIMEN

In the past, most hormone replacement therapy to manage menopause consisted of taking estrogen for part of the month and progesterone for part of the month. Many physicians prefer this alternating hormone regimen for women with intact uteruses because of the increased risk of endometrial cancer when using "unopposed estrogen" (estrogen given alone without progesterone). Estrogen accelerates the buildup of the endometrial lining; progesterone causes sloughing of the endometrial lining, otherwise known as menstruation.

The most commonly used estrogen is conjugated estrogen (Premarin), made from purified urine of pregnant horses. Another option, estradiol (Estrace), is chemically synthesized; although it is not "natural," estradiol is chemically identical to the estrogen produced by your ovaries.

Natural estrogens occurring in plants (phytoestrogens) are sometimes used for menopausal women. They are somewhat chemically different from your own estrogen and may not work in exactly the same way in your body. For example, plant estrogens may not protect against osteoporosis as well as other estrogens.

Most women on HRT take both estrogen and a progestin, generally progesterone. This is usually given as two separate pills, because the progestin is used during only part of the month. The most commonly used progestins are micronized progesterone (Crinone gel) and medroxyprogesterone (Cycrin, Provera, or Amen). They are usually better tolerated by women with migraines than testosterone-based progestins like norethindrone acetate (Aygest).

CONTINUOUS COMBINED THERAPY

Continuous combined hormone therapy is a recent trend in HRT. This involves using both estrogen and a progestin on a daily basis. You take either two separate pills or a combination pill such as PremPro, if it's available in the dosage your physician recommends.

In the summer of 1998 a new transdermal patch delivering continuous combined hormonal therapy was approved by the FDA. The CombiPatch continuously delivers both estrogen and progesterone, but it's still so new I haven't had enough feedback from patients to be able to determine its usefulness in menopausal migraineurs.

DELIVERY FORMS OF HRT

Hormone replacement therapy can be given in pill form, in injectable form, or through the skin. The transdermal form of estrogen—an adhesive-backed patch that's changed every few days—has become extremely popular. Common brand names include Estraderm, Vivelle, Climara, and FemPatch, and there are others. Transdermal estrogen preparation results in smoother blood levels of estrogen because it is continuously absorbed, thus avoiding the hormonal fluctuations that can precipitate migraines.

Conjugated estrogens are the most common form of replacement estrogen prescribed and are given in pill form. Some women develop more migraines on conjugated estrogens and do better with the chemically synthesized estradiol, available as a pill, a transdermal patch, or an injection. Phytoestrogens, which may not be as potent as other forms of estrogen, are available in pill form and in creams.

Estrogen is also available in a vaginal cream and is often used for symptoms associated with vaginal-wall thinning—namely, decreased lubrication and uncomfortable intercourse due to increased friction. However, the vaginal cream does not raise estrogen blood levels as effectively as do other forms of estrogen supplementation.

CONTINUOUS ESTROGEN THERAPY

With our current understanding of how estrogen relates to migraine, the ideal estrogen regimen for migraine sufferers would be continuous estrogen therapy. Indeed, studies have found that menopausal migraine sufferers most frequently report headaches during the days they were *off* estrogen. Most migraineurs seem to fare better on transdermal estrogen, which delivers smoother and more consistent blood levels than pills.

Trista, forty-six, a patient of mine for several years, had always been prone to premenstrual migraines. When she became perimenopausal, her headaches went from bad to worse. Fortunately, however, she has been extremely successful in controlling her migraines by using an estrogen patch for the three days prior to her menstrual period. "This time of the month has gone from being nightmarish to being tolerable," Trista told me. "The patch is the perfect way to get medication. And when you take a shower, you just pull it off and stick it on the bathroom mirror."

A recent study illustrates why continuous estrogen therapy has become the regimen of choice for menopausal migraineurs. The study involved twenty-eight menopausal women, sixteen of whom had a history of severe menstrual migraine during their childbearing years, twelve of whom had no history whatsoever of migraine. All the women were taking continuous estrogen replacement at the beginning of the study. Each woman was given a single monthly injection of estradiol (Depo Estradiol), the chemically synthesized form of estrogen. Blood levels of estradiol were measured as they gradually declined over four weeks.

All of the sixteen women with a history of migraine developed migraines when their blood levels had dropped to less than 50 picograms per milliliter (pg/ml). The other women did not develop migraine, although their estradiol levels also dropped. The study suggests that keeping estradiol levels at or above 50 pg/ml might protect susceptible women from developing migraines. A continuous estrogen regimen would prevent the drop in estrogen levels that might occur with intermittent estrogen/progesterone therapy. If your estradiol level falls below 50 pg/ml, replacement estrogen might alleviate your menopausal migraines.

(Note: Some women with migraines have been advised to avoid estrogen altogether because occasionally estrogen *causes* their headaches.)

BENEFITS OF HORMONE REPLACEMENT THERAPY

In addition to managing the pain of migraine headaches, estrogen replacement therapy (ERT) offers several other significant health benefits. It can alleviate the menopausal symptoms of hot flashes and night sweats as well as vaginal dryness. It protects against osteoporosis (softening of the bones), a serious, common, and potentially debilitating problem among aging women.

What's more, cholesterol levels—increasingly important as women age and lose their protective hormones—are positively affected by estrogen. Estrogen lowers the levels of LDL (or "bad") cholesterol and elevates the levels of HDL (or "good") cholesterol. Unopposed estrogen does a better job of raising HDL levels than combined estrogen therapy. (It is not, however, as effective at lowering cholesterol as targeted medications such as Zocor, Lipitor, or Mevacor.)

Estrogen may also prevent heart disease. In several observational studies (in which a large population is identified and observed over the years, without being subjected to any experiment) estrogen supplementation appeared to play a protective role. In such studies, women on estrogen exhibited lower rates of heart disease than women not on estrogen. (However, there is one caveat: In studies of women who already had heart disease before they entered menopause, estrogen failed to prevent further cardiac problems.)

The HERS (Heart and Estrogen/Progestin Replacement Study), a randomized trial of nearly 2,800 women, led by researchers Deborah Grady, M.D., of the University of California, San Francisco, and William Applegate, M.D., of the University of Tennessee, along with eighteen medical centers nationwide, was designed to look at whether combination therapy is superior to placebo in preventing heart attacks. In the first clinical trial (of women with a history of cardiac ailments), HERS investigators found that combined estrogen and progestin therapy increased the risk of gallbladder disease and blood clots in the legs and lungs. There is some preliminary evidence of cardiac benefit from combined HRT, but results are not yet fully conclusive. Results of this important study should be available in 1999.

Some studies indicate estrogen may protect against colon cancer and possibly against Alzheimer's disease as well. Interestingly, there is no clear evidence that replacement estrogen either increases or decreases risk of stroke. This is somewhat surprising, given the increased risk of stroke seen in premenopausal women on estrogen-containing oral contraceptives.

THE RISKS OF HRT

In addition to the benefits, you should be aware that continuous estrogen therapy—taken daily and without a break—does carry significant risks. In a study spanning three years, reported in the *Journal of the American Medical Association* (*JAMA*) in 1995, one-third of the women taking "unopposed estrogen" developed precancerous lesions of the endometrium, or uterine lining. By contrast, precancerous lesions occurred in less than 1 percent of the women studied who were on the combined therapy of estrogen plus progestogen. This is why most physicians prefer combined therapy. (Of course, if you no longer have a uterus, continuous estrogen therapy presents no uterine risk and is likely to benefit you in terms of migraine relief.)

Whether you are on continuous or alternating estrogen replacement therapy, you do need to know that estrogen supplementation increases the risk of breast cancer. A study of women on long-term estrogen therapy published in *The Lancet* in 1997 showed that these women had a 1.35 times greater chance of developing breast cancer than women not on any form of estrogen. Another related problem with estrogen vis-à-vis breast cancer is that it increases the density of breast tissue, thus making the interpretation of mammograms more problematic. An incipient lump might be more easily missed and might progress to a more serious stage when finally caught.

What's more, because one of its side effects is the proliferation of the endometrial lining, which is associated with uterine cancer, the use of estrogen will increase your chances of needing a hysterectomy. It will also double your lifetime risk of needing gallbladder surgery, as well as increasing your prospects of developing blood clots in your veins or lungs.

SHOULD YOU CONSIDER HRT?

Despite the risks, most experts do recommend continuous unopposed estrogen therapy for the treatment of problematic menopausal migraines. Before signing on, however, patients should receive a full discussion of the risks. What's more, dosages should be individualized for you by your physician, based on your medical situation, symptoms, and family history. If you still have your uterus, you should receive frequent gynecologic checkups. (Depending on your risk factors, exams could be recommended anywhere from every two months to twice a year.) Some experts advocate frequent uterine ultrasounds and endometrial biopsies as well.

Others recommend simultaneous continuous estrogen and continuous progestin therapy. While combined continuous therapy does protect the uterine lining, two problems are associated with it. It can produce unpredictable bleeding in some women, which is somewhat like having periods without any warning of when they'll begin. About half of the women on continuous combined therapy stop bleeding altogether; a few spot continuously. A more significant problem, however, is that while the progestins serve to protect migraineurs from developing cancer, many women experience migraine headaches as a side effect of taking progestins. Some women on combined continuous therapy even develop *daily* migraines.

Because of these problems, sometimes physicians prescribe unopposed estrogen for three or four months, then withdraw the estrogen and give progestin by itself. This will result in a migraine *and* a menstrual period. But at least you only have to deal with it three or four times a year and can predict (and control) when it will occur.

WHAT IF YOU NEED HRT BUT FEAR WORSE MIGRAINES?

If you are hesitant or fearful about taking HRT, then you might consider opting for the lowest possible dose of medication to see if your symptoms improve. Recent studies have revealed that even doses as low as 0.3 milligrams of esterified estrogen tablets, such as Estratab, can protect women from osteoporosis, so it's possible that even with a dose that low (about half the usual starting dose of estrogen), your migraines might also improve.

The only way you can really know if HRT will improve or worsen your migraines is to try it. As with many medications, you will need to give it an adequate trial of at least two to three months (you and your physician can determine exactly how long). If your menopausal symptoms improve and your migraines are no worse, you may want to continue the medications. But if it makes your headaches worse, you may wish to discontinue the medication and consider alternative methods of managing your menopausal symptoms, such as blood-pressure medications, which are sometimes used.

One note of caution: Don't suddenly drop any medication without first consulting your physician. You'll feel much better if you taper the medication down rather than abruptly stop it and throw your body into a tailspin, which would likely include symptoms of menopause, such as hot flashes.

There is also evidence to indicate that you can delay hormone replacement therapy until your sixties and still derive a significant benefit in terms of osteoporosis prevention, while avoiding the cons of HRT during your younger years.

SHOULD YOU CONTINUE YOUR REGULAR MIGRAINE MEDICATIONS DURING MENOPAUSE?

If you're currently on migraine medication and entering menopause, or if you've had success with a particular form of migraine treatment in the past—before you started experiencing menopausal symptoms—you may wonder if you can continue to take it. The answer is, usually you can. However, I've found that for some of my menstrually associated migraine patients, the treatments that worked in the past are no longer as effective when they approach menopause.

For example, Grace, forty-nine, had occasional migraines, easily managed with a medication that combines aspirin, caffeine, butalbital, and codeine (Fiorinal with codeine). Then she hit her late forties and developed ferocious monthly premenstrual migraines. These became worse and worse, until she had a continuous headache for two weeks out of each month, starting midcycle and ending after her period. Grace tried several preventative medications for migraine, to no avail. She tried all the triptans, which were effective, but because they're designed for intermittent use she didn't want to take them daily for two weeks. Even though she is still menstruating fairly regularly, I am convinced that Grace is entering menopause, which is causing the migraines. Grace's gynecologist and I are considering putting her on hormone replacement therapy to help her situation.

Still, while HRT may reduce the number and severity of migraines, it is unlikely to make you headache-free. More than likely, you'll continue to need another medication strategy for managing your migraines.

What's more, as you age, you'll have new medication issues to contend with. For example, postmenopausal women are more prone than menstruating women to develop heart disease, which is, after all, the number-one cause of death in older women. If you have heart disease, you won't be able to take some of the now-standard "workhorse" triptan medications, like sumatriptan (Imitrex), or ergot medications (such as Ergomar or Ergostat). (This is because triptans constrict cardiac and brain blood vessels, while ergots constrict blood vessels in those areas and many others as well). (Read more about medications in Chapter 7.) However, the good news about aging is that as you get older, the incidence of migraine in women decreases.

WILL HYSTERECTOMY HELP?

In a complete hysterectomy, your uterus, ovaries, and Fallopian tubes are removed, resulting in surgical menopause. A simple hysterectomy is surgery in which only your uterus is taken. Removing the uterus doesn't alter hormone levels and should have no effect on your migraines, except that when you no longer have periods, it becomes harder to tell when your hormones are cycling. But a complete hysterectomy can make your headaches worse because surgical menopause divorces you from the ebb and flow (and protection) of your hormones. If your menstrual headaches worsen during perimenopause, you might conclude that a hysterectomy might eliminate the problem. But this is far from true.

Studies have shown that women migraineurs who experience natural menopause fare far better than women who go through surgical menopause. For example, a 1993 study found that of women who went through natural menopause, only 9 percent suffered worse migraines, with 67 percent showing improvement and 24 percent exhibiting no change in migraine frequency or intensity. But among women who underwent surgical menopause (complete hysterectomy), only 33 percent noted improvement of migraine, while fully 67 percent found that their migraines had worsened.

However, if you need a hysterectomy for other reasons, don't hesitate to have it performed because of your migraines.

IF YOU'VE HAD A HYSTERECTOMY

Many women have had hysterectomies before they ever reached menopause or the perimenopausal period. If only your uterus was removed, you will still go through menopause, and you will still need to make a decision about hormone replacement therapy. Since you no longer have periods, it will be more difficult to tell when you are entering menopause. Blood tests will help your physician gauge your hormone levels.

Without a uterus, you will not need progestins and can be safely managed with continuous estrogen therapy, the form of HRT recommended for menopausal migraineurs.

If you had a complete hysterectomy, you are most likely already on a regimen of estrogen replacement therapy or, at a minimum, osteoporosis-prevention therapy. If migraines do not respond to usual migraine treatment, an adjustment in your estrogen dose may help.

MIGRAINES AND MENOPAUSE

Menopause has never been an easy period in a woman's life. Along with the curtailment of your reproductive capabilities, there are emotional, physical, and psychological aspects to contend with. If you suffer from migraines, this difficult time is made more so. However, the bright side of the picture is that now is the best time ever to be a woman addressing the once-taboo topics of menopause and migraine. As members of the groundbreaking baby boom generation approach and enter menopause, there is greater openness about discussing medical matters with friends, coworkers, family, and medical professionals. Baby boomers are more proactive in seeking out the best care available and, therefore, more likely to find real relief for migraines.

Also, during this past decade, the drug companies have been busy designing better, quicker, and more effective medications for you. I'll take a hard look at these new drugs as well as the old "tried-and-true" migraine medications in the next chapter.

CHAPTER
7

Medications That Make a Difference

WHAT'S UP, DOC?

You may think you've tried every conceivable medication for migraine, but more than likely there are some you've never even heard of. More medications exist today for the prevention and treatment of migraine than ever before, with more delivery options—everything from shots you can give yourself at your home or work for fast relief to quick-acting nasal sprays to time-release patches to the old faithful pills. As medical research has gained a greater understanding of the physiology of migraine, the pharmaceutical companies have responded by developing new products in record numbers.

These new medications have revolutionized the treatment of migraine. While nothing has yet been invented to *eliminate* your migraine tendency altogether, what is available can decrease the frequency and severity of your headaches. Rather than just blocking pain, the newer medications can eradicate a migraine attack, including nausea and other symptoms. In some cases the meds make it possible for women to be pain-free, fully present for themselves, their families, and their jobs. And more new medications are in the pipeline and due out over the next few years.

This book is the first to survey the entire field of migraine medicines, analyzing their overall effectiveness while taking a hard look at potential side effects. I'll discuss the possible interactions of various medications with one another and whether you can use these drugs singly or in combination with others over the long haul. And I'll survey what we physicians call "off-label-use" drugs, that is, medications that are accepted and commonly prescribed by the medical community but have not been specifically approved for migraine treatment by the Food and Drug Administration (FDA). Being aware of these medications will expand your knowledge base further and may present options to suggest to your physician. Once you and your doctor come up with an appropriate regimen, you may happily join the ranks of migraineurs who have become virtually headache-free.

As a chronic migraineur myself, I can now go for four to five months at a time between migraines with my present preventative regimen of lisinopril (Zestril or Prinivil). Previously, I experienced one to three migraines a month.

SUFFERING IN VAIN

Despite all these powerful and liberating new medications, the majority of migraine sufferers still use only over-the-counter medications to manage their headache pain. While these OTC drugs can work to combat mild migraines, they're no match for the mind-splitting, excruciating variety. They simply do not provide adequate relief for the majority of migraine attacks.

In my view, it's not right for you to suffer unnecessarily if prescription medications that can help are available. With more than fifty nonnarcotic medications on the market for the treatment and prevention of migraines, it's likely that one or more of them will work for you. These pharmaceutical breakthroughs not only can improve your quality of life as a migraineur, but they can have positive repercussions on your career. By slashing your downtime, they'll improve your likelihood of finding a more stable and fulfilling work situation, with a greater chance for advancement and pay hikes. As I counsel my patients, no one benefits when you suffer in vain.

TREATMENT OF ACUTE MIGRAINE ATTACK

ANALGESICS

Almost everyone is familiar with analgesic painkillers. Most migraineurs have at one time used over-the-counter analgesic remedies to try to manage their headaches. In fact, an estimated 114 million Americans used nonprescription pain relievers in 1996, according to *American Demographics* magazine. About 69 percent of all over-the-counter analgesics are taken for headaches. (Of course, not all of these headaches were migraines.)

Analgesics vary considerably in strength, ranging from the aspirin you can buy in any pharmacy or convenience store to the prescription-strength variety, including controlled medications such as narcotics, for which you may need a special prescription or an office visit. Until recently, OTC analgesics and narcotics were the mainstay of treatments for acute migraine attacks. But with the advent of new migraine-specific medications, they're used less frequently.

SIMPLE ANALGESICS
Simple analgesics are nonnarcotic analgesic medications such as aspirin and acetaminophen (Tylenol), which can help some women with mild migraine. (Even if you've never had a migraine before, it is possible to have a mild migraine. Migraine is defined by the characteristics of the headache symptoms, such as one-sided pain and nausea, not necessarily by the intensity of the pain.)

But don't assume that because they're simple analgesics—

"only" aspirin or acetaminophen (Tylenol)—they're benign. In fact, even simple analgesics can cause problems and should not be overused. Excessive use of aspirin, for example, can cause microscopic bleeding from the stomach and can aggravate an ulcer or lead to anemia. Similarly, overreliance on acetaminophen can result in liver damage. Chronic excessive use of either or both aspirin and acetaminophen over many years can cause kidney damage.

COMPOUND ANALGESICS

Compound analgesics are medications containing aspirin or acetaminophen in combination with other ingredients, often caffeine. Some are over-the-counter medications, while others require a prescription. For example, two frequently prescribed compound analgesics contain mild doses of a barbiturate along with aspirin or acetaminophen and caffeine; therefore, you need a doctor's prescription to obtain them in the United States. The first medication, Fioricet, is a combination of acetaminophen, caffeine, and butalbital, and the second, Fiorinal, is composed of aspirin, caffeine, and butalbital. (Prescriptions of Fioricet and Fiorinal are also available with codeine.)

Listed below are the generic components of several popular combination analgesics with their brand names in parentheses:

- aspirin, acetaminophen, caffeine (Excedrin)
- aspirin, butalbital, caffeine (Fiorinal, Fiortal, or Lanorinal)
- acetaminophen, butalbital, caffeine (Esgic, Fioricet, or Isocet)
- acetaminophen, caffeine (Phrenilin, Sedapap)
- dichloralphenazone, isometheptene, and acetaminophen (Midrin, Duradrin, Midchlor)

Midrin is a nonnarcotic combination analgesic that contains mildly vasoconstrictive (blood-vessel–constricting) agents. It's often effective in treating an acute migraine.

Midrin, Duradrin, and Midchlor all contain the same ingredients but must be avoided if you have glaucoma, heart disease, liver disease, kidney disease, or uncontrolled high blood pressure. Do not take acetaminophen with them, as they already contain some and doubling your dose will increase the risk of liver damage, which has been associated with acetaminophen overuse.

These medications can be very useful for mild to moderate migraine headaches, if taken infrequently. But with frequent use, you not only run the risk of organ damage from excessive aspirin or acetaminophen use, you also risk experiencing rebound headaches.

Never take these drugs preventively. Some migraineurs are so fearful they *might* develop a headache that they take an analgesic pill in case. But since analgesics don't prevent headaches, this is a misuse of the medicine. They should only be taken to relieve pain you already have.

NARCOTIC ANALGESICS

Narcotic analgesics are sometimes used to treat headache, although less frequently than in the past, since the advent of migraine-specific medications has made them unnecessary. Narcotic analgesics often contain a simple analgesic (such as aspirin or acetaminophen) in addition to the narcotic. Examples of some narcotics are codeine, hydrocodone, oxycodone, propoxyphene, and morphine. Here are some narcotics with their prominent brand names:

- hydrocodon and acetaminophen (Anexsia, Panacet, Lortab, Vicodin)
- acetaminophen, oxycodone (Tylox, Percocet)
- aspirin, oxycodone (Percodan)
- acetaminophen, propoxyphene napsylate (Darvocet)
- meperidine HCI (Demerol)
- pentazocine (Talwin)
- acetaminophen, codeine (Tylenol #3)

I'm concerned that some of the newer medications—which have been touted as nonaddictive, even though they are semisynthetic opioids—may in fact be addictive in susceptible individuals. Examples include tramadol HCl (Ultram) and butorphanol tartrate (Stadol).

Some adverse effects of opioid narcotic analgesics include:

- constipation
- loss of appetite
- nausea
- sedation
- mood changes
- anxiety
- urinary retention
- itching or skin rash
- occasionally, worsening of headache pain

"My doctor has known me for years, and I have never abused narcotics," you may say. "They've always worked for my headaches. Why can't I just keep using them?" Maybe you can and *should* continue using narcotics on an as-needed basis. But there may be valid reasons for discontinuing these medications.

Your doctor may observe that you're getting headaches more frequently and want to help you avoid rebound headache, which can be caused by narcotic analgesics. Maybe your laboratory tests have revealed early evidence of kidney problems, and continuing analgesics could be putting you in jeopardy. Or you may also have other symptoms that could represent complications caused by the narcotic.

When narcotic medications are used chronically, they encourage your brain to produce more opiate receptors. With more opiate receptors, you require more medication to block them and therefore block the pain. This sets up a vicious cycle in which you continually need more and more medication. In addition to being addictive, narcotic analgesics can cause rebound headache. This is why doctors recommend that narcotic analgesics be used infrequently.

No doubt about it: Narcotics are appropriate in some situations. One example is the woman whose regular migraine medications work on her for other migraines but not on the migraine that descends upon her right before or during her period. Narcotic analgesics for this monthly menstrual headache would be appropriate.

But if you haven't tried the newer migraine-specific medications, keep an open mind. They may work much better for your headache than the narcotic you've been using all these years.

NONSTEROIDAL ANTI-INFLAMMATORY DRUGS

Steroids have limited use in the management of migraine because of their complicated and potentially severe side effects. Nonsteroidal anti-inflammatory drugs (NSAID's), however, have far fewer adverse effects and thus are much safer to use.

You can find some common NSAID's over the counter including ibuprofen (Motrin, Advil), ketoprofen (Actron), naproxen sodium (Aleve, Anaprox), and aspirin. There are many other prescription NSAID's that can be useful in treating mild to moderate migraine, either as "adjunctive medication" (given with something else) or on their own. One study showed that flurbiprofen alone was adequate to abort acute migraine attacks in 30 percent of cases. Naproxen sodium has also been used effectively to halt acute attacks.

NSAID's are especially useful with the mixed headache, one with characteristics of both a migraine and a tension-type headache. On the negative side, however, some experts believe that NSAID's may create rebound headaches. However, this problem appears to occur far less frequently than with analgesics.

Sometimes an acute migraine attack can be aborted by using high-dose anti-inflammatories or antinausea medications. Studies have demonstrated the benefits of taking naproxen sodium or flurbiprofen at the onset of a migraine. The combination of aspirin and metoclopramide, an antinausea medication, has also been shown to be effective in aborting migraine attacks in some women.

ERGOT-BASED MEDICATIONS

Introduced to treat migraines in 1926, ergotamine—which is extracted from the ergot fungus that grows on rye—is one of the oldest migraine medications still in use. Ergot medications are available in oral, rectal, nasal, and injectable forms. They include

- ergonovine maleate (Ergotrate maleate, injectable)
- ergotamine tartrate (Ergomar, Ergostat)
- dihydroergotamine (DHE-45, injectable; Migranal, nasal spray)
- ergotamine tartrate and caffeine (Cafergot, Ercaf, or Wigraine)

Ergot medications often cause nausea but are frequently effective at aborting a migraine attack. Dihydroergotamine, which works rapidly because it is administered as a nasal spray or by injection, is somewhat less likely to cause nausea.

Women who are pregnant cannot use ergots because they act as vasoconstrictors of the blood supply to the placenta and might inhibit the fetus's circulation and normal development.

NEW KIDS ON THE BLOCK: THE TRIPTANS

The triptans have provided an exciting breakthrough and a welcome relief in the field of migraine treatment. The first triptan, sumatriptan (Imitrex), was introduced in the American market in 1993 in injectable form and has since been embraced by many migraineurs. Pharmaceutical experts report that this medication alone skyrocketed sales of prescription migraine medications in the United States by nearly 61 percent from 1995 to 1996—up to a total of $639 million. In 1996 Imitrex became available as a tablet, and the following year it was introduced as a nasal spray. Imitrex was followed by three more triptans in 1998: zolmitriptan (Zomig), naratriptan (Amerge), and rizatriptan (Maxalt).

"I love that Imitrex!" said Dana, fifty-four, a patient who has suffered from migraines since age ten. "Unlike Cafergot, Stadol, or Demerol, Imitrex allows me to function. The pain often goes away in fifteen minutes, with no downtime."

Pat, forty, a migraine sufferer since the age of nine, said: "My migraines are severe. On a scale of one to ten, with one being mild, my headaches are nines and tens or they're off the scale. Thanks to Fiorinal and Imitrex, the pain is down to a three-to-five level. I can deal with that. For the last two years, Imitrex has relieved all but one big migraine."

One key benefit of the triptans is their ability to act quickly. Studies of the effectiveness of the sumatriptan (Imitrex) tablet showed about a 71 percent rate of headache relief at four hours, with relief defined as "mild or no pain." With an injection of sumatriptan (Imitrex), 70 percent of migraineurs showed relief after sixty minutes, and fully 49 percent were pain-free. Studies of rizatriptan (Maxalt) showed 37 percent relief at one hour and 67 percent at two hours. Studies of zolmitriptan (Zomig) resulted in a 62 to 65 percent rate of relief after two hours, with 27 percent of subjects being pain-free.

A major problem with many headache remedies—including the triptans—is that the headache comes back once the medicine wears off. However, studies of naratriptan (Amerge) have revealed that for 81 percent of those who responded to the medication, headache didn't recur over a twenty-four-hour period. But there is a trade-off: Naratriptan (Amerge) does not work as rapidly as do the other triptans. Studies of both zolmitriptan and sumatriptan have demonstrated their efficacy in treating menstrual migraines.

Antimigraine Medications: Not Painkillers
What is unique about the triptans is that they work very specifically as antimigraine medications. They are not pain

medications and will not do battle with pains in other body parts. By contrast, analgesics target all pain, wherever its location.

However, the triptans work on *all* migraine symptoms, including nausea and sensitivity to bright lights and loud sounds. Triptans work within the wall of the blood vessels in the brain, and possibly within the brain itself, on a type of serotonin receptor. Experts believe they decrease neurotransmitter activity and "turn off" the migraine.

Unlike ergotamine or isometheptene, dichloralphenazone, and acetaminophen—which must be taken at the beginning of a headache in order to be fully effective—triptan medications can be taken at any time during the attack.

Forms of Triptans

Delivery forms of triptans vary from brand to brand. As discussed, sumatriptan is available as a tablet, a nasal spray, and in injectable form for a subcutaneous injection. (A subcutaneous injection, just under the skin, is not as complex to learn as an intramuscular injection, and many patients have learned to self-administer.)

Rizatriptan is uniquely available in a mint-flavored wafer that melts in the mouth. This formulation was created especially for migraineurs who become nauseated when swallowing tablets or who need to take medication discreetly or when a glass of water is not available. A standard tablet formulation of rizatriptan is also available.

Zolmitriptan is presently available only in tablet form, but a nasal spray and a rapidly dissolving tablet are in development. Still other triptans (eletriptan and frovatriptan) are in the testing phase and should be released soon.

The triptan medications as a whole have been very useful for migraine sufferers who cannot tolerate other medications or have not found them effective. If one triptan doesn't work, another may. Also, one may work faster or more effectively for you. Consult with your doctor to try to find the one that's best for you.

Side Effects of Triptans

As with all medications, triptans have side effects. Here are the most common:

- flushing of the face or throat
- burning sensations in the head, throat, or chest
- chest tightness
- tingling in the face
- head rush

These side effects occur more often with the injected form of medication than with oral forms. A worsening of nausea can occur with any triptan, but this happens infrequently. The nasal spray can leave a bitter aftertaste in your mouth.

Not everyone can take triptans. Because they constrict cardiac blood vessels by as much as 10 percent in diameter, they should not be taken by individuals with heart disease, peripheral vascular disease, uncontrolled high blood pressure, or the rare forms of migraine known as basilar migraine or hemiplegic migraine.

A few notes of caution: Triptans should not be taken if you are currently using an MAO-inhibitor antidepressant. (MAO inhibitors are a class of medications that work through a complicated series of events in the brain to prevent migraine. They include phenelzine (Nardil) and isocarboxazide (Marplan) but are used infrequently because of their potential for serious side effects, such as a hypertensive crisis, which can be fatal.) What's more, because both triptans and ergots are vasoconstrictive drugs (meaning that they shrink the diameter of the vessels), they should not be taken together. Instead, you should allow a twenty-four-hour gap between the use of an ergot and the use of a triptan. Finally, rizatriptan (Maxalt) should be taken at a reduced dose if you are also taking the medication propanolol (Inderal).

The Cost of Triptans

While the prices of the triptan medications vary somewhat, they're all more expensive than analgesics and the other medications discussed in this chapter. One triptan pill might set you back fifteen dollars, while a single injection could run you forty-two dollars or more. Nonetheless, many women consider them a bargain at any price for their effectiveness in eliminating migraines.

However, let me emphasize that triptans are not magic bullets for everyone. Jennifer, thirty-eight, who has had migraines since adolescence, told me: "For many people the new meds are wonderful, but none have worked for me. All the publicity helps people to learn about them, but on the other hand, it make the general public less compassionate for those of us who don't get positive results. We're often treated like there must be something mentally wrong with us if the new medications don't work." My recommendation for women like Jennifer is to work with her doctor to determine if there are any medications she hasn't considered and give them a try.

PREVENTATIVE MEDICATIONS

For the majority of sufferers, migraines occur once or twice a month. If your migraines respond to acute therapy, no further medication is necessary. For some women, however, headaches occur more frequently, or those two monthly headaches are severe and last for several days. When frequent or severe headaches occur, a medication taken on a daily basis to prevent migraine may be useful. It is sometimes possible to suppress the migraine attacks entirely; it is usually possible to at least decrease the number and severity of attacks.

Preventative medications are often selected on the basis of your overall health. For example, if you have a tendency toward high blood pressure, there are migraine preventative medications that are also high blood pressure medications, such as beta blockers.

Beta Blockers
Propanolol was one of the first beta-blocker medications used in migraine prevention. Researchers suspect they work

in the brain itself, probably on neurotransmitters known as catecholamines, to prevent migraine.

There are many beta blockers, some of which are ineffective in preventing migraine. However the following have a strong track record in preventing migraine: Metoprolol (Lopressor), nadolol (Corgard), timolol (Blocadren), atenolol (Tenormin), and propanolol (Inderal).

Beta blockers can limit your exercise tolerance by slowing your heart rate. Other adverse effects may include fatigue, depression, dizziness, sleep disturbances, or abnormal dreams. Individuals with asthma, emphysema, congestive heart failure, cardiac-conduction defects, or peripheral vascular disease cannot use beta blockers. Many diabetics cannot either. Check with your physician.

What if your blood pressure is already on the low side? Will a beta blocker lower it still further? It may, although this is not necessarily a problem, as long as you can tolerate it. You may feel a little light-headed, or it might not bother you at all. Balance out this side effect with how well it works to suppress your migraines. Also, consider the fact that although one beta blocker doesn't work for you, another might.

Calcium Channel Blockers

Another type of blood-pressure medication used for migraine prevention is the calcium channel blocker. Calcium channel blockers do not affect the overall calcium level in your body or in your bloodstream. Instead, they work very specifically at a channel within the blood-vessel wall that lets calcium through, blocking entry of calcium into that cell. Abnormal calcium channels can be associated with migraine in some patients.

There are several kinds of calcium channels, which have different biological effects. Researchers are fairly certain that calcium channel blockers work in the brain to prevent migraine rather than in the actual peripheral blood-vessel calcium channels.

Calcium channel blockers include verapamil (Calan, Isoptin, Covera, Verelan), diltiazem (Cardizem, Dilacor, Tiazac), nicardipine (Cardene), and nifedipine (Adalat, Procardia). Procardia causes headaches in about 40 percent of the people who take it; hence it's no longer widely used by migraineurs.

Calcium channel blockers are fairly well tolerated. Common adverse effects are constipation, ankle swelling, nausea, mild headache, dizziness, or low blood pressure. Some women also experience weight gain—probably from constipation. Calcium channel blockers cannot be used if you experience certain heart-rhythm problems, such as bradycardia or sick-sinus syndrome, or if you are already on a beta blocker. Safety in pregnancy and during lactation has not been established.

One disadvantage of the calcium channel blockers is time. They take up to eight weeks to become fully effective in your system, whereas most of the other preventative medications require only two to six weeks to provide full benefits.

Clonidine

Clonidine (Catapres) is another type of blood-pressure medication that is used for migraine prevention. A centrally acting antihypertensive, it works in the brain to control blood pressure. It is also used to treat various chronic pain syndromes as well as migraines. Clonidine can cause sedation, dizziness, depression, or anxiety.

Divalproex Sodium

An antiepileptic medication, divalproex sodium (Depakote) has received FDA approval for prevention of migraine. Divalproex sodium is thought to work on a neurotransmitter called gamma-aminobutyric acid (GABA). One study revealed that migraine sufferers had lower levels of salivary GABA than nonmigraine sufferers, and those levels drop even further during a migraine attack.

Divalproex sodium can't be used if you have liver disease. Your doctor may want to monitor your blood while you are on divalproex sodium to make sure there is no significant increase in liver enzymes. And the medication should be used with caution in women of childbearing age because it can cause birth defects if taken during pregnancy, especially in early pregnancy. Be sure you are using an effective method of contraception if you take divalproex sodium.

You should be aware that about 10 percent of the women who take this medication will experience some weight gain. In my experience, though, this weight generally drops off after you stop taking the medication. For most women, any weight gained from taking divalproex sodium is not as hard to lose as weight gained from other medications (such as steroids or tricyclic antidepressants).

Other side effects that can occur with divalproex sodium include constipation, mild gastric distress, dry mouth, leg cramps, abnormal dreams, or tremor.

Tricyclic Antidepressants
Tricyclic antidepressants have been used for migraine prevention as well as other chronic ailments. If your physician prescribes a tricyclic antidepressant, it does not necessarily mean he thinks you are suffering from depression.

These medications are believed to act on the brain chemical known as noradrenaline. Only amitriptyline (Elavil) has shown consistent efficacy in formal studies as a migraine preventative. But nortriptyline (Pamelor, Aventyl) and doxepin (Sinequan) are often found to be effective clinically and are also commonly prescribed.

Amitriptyline has more serotonin activity than the other tricyclic antidepressants. Of the three, doxepin tends to be the most sedating, and nortriptyline the least. Other common adverse effects include constipation, weight gain, dry mouth, and nausea.

Heather, thirty-five, was plagued by severe migraines about once a week, lasting for a day or two. She was often awakened at night by pounding pain and nausea, making it difficult, if not impossible, to take a pill for her migraine. Since starting on a nightly preventive dose of 25 milligrams of amitriptyline, Heather has had only one or two mild headaches a month, without the debilitating nausea. These migraines she treats with naproxen sodium (Aleve).

Tricyclic antidepressants cannot be used if you have certain cardiac arrhythmias, and they should be used with caution in the elderly. Tricyclics also lower the seizure threshold and should be used on epileptics only with your physician's approval and only if you are on an effective antiepilepsy regimen.

SSRI Antidepressants

The newer antidepressant medications are in the class called "serotonin selective reuptake inhibitors" (SSRI's) and are often targeted as potential headache medications. You've probably heard of fluoxetine (Prozac), which falls within this category. Other examples of SSRI's are sertraline (Zoloft) and paroxetine (Paxil). These medications work primarily at the 5HT2 receptor, which is not important in acute migraine pain. Researchers have achieved mixed results when studying the effectiveness of these SSRI antidepressants in treating migraine.

Venlafaxine (Effexor), another form of SSRI, has also shown some effectiveness. This medication acts on both serotonin and noradrenaline. Serzone (nefazadone) has also been successfully used in the prevention of migraine.

Colleen, thirty-nine, a patient who was diagnosed with migraines at age twenty-two, said, "I don't respond well to abortive medications, but the new antidepressants have worked wonders for me. The change from nortriptyline (Pamelor) to nefazadone (Serzone) has been remarkable. Last year, I had forty-five migraines from January 1 to April 15. This year, with the Serzone, it was down to eighteen."

Many headache specialists feel the SSRI antidepressants are especially effective in migraine if the migraine sufferer is also depressed.

Common adverse effects of these medications are nausea, mild headache, sedation, alteration in sleep cycles, and suppression of the sex drive or an inability to climax.

Methysergide

Methysergide (Sansert), which was approved for migraine treatment in 1959, is still used, although not as widely now that we have so many more attractive options. When other medications fail, it can often suppress chronic migraine.

Because of potentially serious adverse effects (namely, the formation of fibrous tissue around the kidneys, in the heart valves, or in the lungs), methysergide is usually given for six months, followed by a one-month drug "holiday" before it is resumed. If it is given over a longer period, the patient is usually closely monitored with an abdominal MRI every six to twelve months. (Other adverse effects include nausea, dizziness, muscle cramps, drowsiness, weight gain, flushing, nasal congestion, insomnia, or pain or swelling in the extremities.)

Methysergide cannot be taken if you have peripheral vascular disease, heart disease, or ulcers, or if you're pregnant. It should also be avoided if you have high blood pressure that's difficult to control with medication, or if you have a familial tendency to develop fibrosis of organs or tissues.

Although it sounds terrible, methysergide can be extremely useful in pain relief for the severe chronic migraine sufferer who has not fared well with other medicines. Despite its risks, it is very effective. And as long as it's given appropriately and monitored carefully, it can be safe.

A cautionary note: Triptan medications cannot be used in conjunction with methysergide. Ergot medications can be used for acute attacks, but because both drugs are vasoconstrictor agents, using half the usual effective dose is recommended.

Nonsteroidal Anti-Inflammatory Drugs as Preventives

Earlier in the chapter, we looked at how NSAID's can treat acute migraine attacks. Some headache researchers believe

NSAID's are also effective in migraine prevention. Naproxen sodium (Anaprox, Naprelan, Aleve) has been shown to be useful, as has tolfenamic acid, a drug that is marketed in Europe. Ketoprofen (Orudis, Oruvail), mefenamic acid (Ponstel), and fenoprofen (Nalfon) may also be of some use, although study results vary.

Adverse effects of these medications include diarrhea, gastrointestinal discomfort, and erosive gastritis, which can cause bleeding from the stomach and result in anemia. These medications cannot be used if you have kidney or liver disease, active peptic-ulcer disease, aspirin allergy, or if you are taking an anticoagulant medication. Most obstetricians allow the use of NSAID's in early pregnancy but recommend they be discontinued in the fourth month of gestation.

MISCELLANEOUS MEDICATIONS

Cyproheptadine (Periactin) has been used to treat migraines for a long time. It was developed as an antihistamine and has chemical properties similar to those of the tricyclic antidepressants. Cyproheptadine has shown variable results in the few controlled studies that have been done.

Adverse effects include sedation, weight gain, dizziness, dry mouth, and increased appetite. Cyproheptadine is still commonly used for migraine in children because it is safe, and children seem to tolerate the medication with fewer adverse effects than adults.

Gabapentin (Neurontin) is an antiepileptic medication that works on the neurotransmitter GABA. Because divalproex sodium (Depakote) works on GABA to suppress migraines, it has been theorized that other GABA medications might have the same effect. Large-scale trials of gabapentin in migraine prevention are currently under way, and results should be available soon. Clinics reporting success with gabapentin indicate that fairly high doses are required. The primary adverse effect of gabapentin is sedation, therefore it is usually given at night. Because it is not metabolized but is excreted by the body unchanged, it is safe to mix with other medications.

In the past, other antiepileptic medications have been proposed and tried for migraine, including phenytoin (Dilantin) and carbamezepine (Tegretol). These are now seldom used. Other medications have shown higher response rates and fewer adverse effects.

Lithium carbonate (Lithotab, Lithobid) can be quite useful in the treatment of chronic cluster headache and has sometimes been tried in cases of chronic migraines. Large-scale trials have not established a role for lithium in the prevention of migraine.

THE COMPOUNDING PHARMACIST

If your particular medication doesn't come in a form that works for you, it may be possible for your doctor to work with a compounding pharmacist to arrange a delivery mode that you'll find effective. A compounding pharmacist can make a formulation from existing medications. Find out if your pharmacist is a compounding pharmacist; if not, your state board of pharmacy can refer you to the nearest compounding pharmacist in your area. Here in Oregon I work with compounding pharmacists who put an antinausea medication into a topical gel to rub into the skin. This is much more appealing to some of my patients than using a suppository.

It is also possible to put an anti-inflammatory in a cream for massaging directly into the skin. Not only does this avoid the stomach irritation some people get with anti-inflammatories, it also places the medication right where it hurts. There are many other possibilities for solving medication-delivery problems through specially compounded formulations. Ask your doctor about them.

MUSCLE RELAXERS

If you get more than one kind of headache, it may be difficult to distinguish whether a beginning headache is indeed a migraine or some other type of headache. You may even feel yourself getting two headaches at once. If your neck gets tight along with the headache, often a muscle relaxer will be prescribed in addition to migraine medication.

Muscle relaxers commonly used are cyclobenzaprine (Flexeril), metaxolone (Skelaxin), orphenadrine citrate (Norflex), carisoprodol (Soma), methocarbamol (Robaxin), and baclofen (Lioresal). Most of these are sedating. Some seem to diminish in effectiveness after a few weeks of daily use.

Soma (carisoprodol) has been designated a controlled substance in my home state of Oregon because it has become a drug of abuse. Used correctly, however, muscle relaxers can help prevent headache recurrence in those who suffer from mixed headaches.

IS THAT ALL THERE IS?

If this description of migraine medications and possible side effects gives you pause, remember that most medications don't cause side effects in every person. Rarely will you experience every possible side effect that could occur. In most cases, you won't contract any side effect.

If you've tried most of these and haven't found an effective remedy for your migraine, or if you'd simply like to try a nonpharmaceutical approach for freeing yourself of migraine pain, keep reading. In the next chapter, I'll lay out the nontraditional routes to surviving and triumphing over your migraine problem.

CHAPTER
8

Alternative Remedies

Maybe you're having migraines for the first time, and before signing on to a regimen of prescription drugs, you'd like to do everything possible to ward them off with exercise, lifestyle changes, and alternative remedies. Or perhaps you're pregnant and seeking natural antidotes for migraine to protect the safety of your unborn child. Or drugs work for you but you'd simply like to explore alternatives to reduce your reliance on powerful and costly medications.

Whatever your motivation, in this chapter I'll examine nonmedication and alternative remedies that may help prevent your migraines—or at least make them more manageable. I'll look at well-accepted forms of nonmedication therapy such as massage, physical therapy, and old-fashioned exercise that could help tackle your migraines as well as boost your overall wellness. And I'll address less well-tested forms of treatment for migraine such as chiropractic manipulation, acupuncture, hypnosis, aromatherapy, and herb and vitamin supplementation. Some of these approaches may prove to be the quickest way for you to achieve real relief, or they may simply complement your existing regimen.

Bear in mind that just as with prescription drugs, not every alternative approach will suit everyone. Before trying any of these remedies, check in with your doctor for advice; if you do decide to try one of these alternative remedies, be sure to put your doctor in the loop so that he can factor it into your overall program of migraine care.

Physicians like myself have been slow to accept some of these alternative remedies for migraine—and with good reason. Many of these programs or substances are hard to recommend because they haven't been through the rigors of scientific testing that could deem them both safe and effective. Though I urge you to be cautious and not accept quick-fix claims at face value without doing your own digging, I certainly do not discount alternative approaches altogether. In fact, while more study needs to be done into a number of them, I am the first to say that a combination of medication, lifestyle changes, and alternative remedies can yield *better results* for the management of migraine than medication alone.

HANDS-ON METHODS FOR TACKLING MIGRAINE

There are several physical techniques that may help you wage the good fight with your migraines. Arguably the best known and accepted is massage therapy, in which the muscles in your neck, upper back, and often your entire body are massaged for the purpose of muscle relaxation and enhanced circulation. Physical therapy—in which a trained therapist provides a variety of strengthening exercises and methods of muscle relaxation—is yet another technique that you may find helpful. Other forms of physical treatment include chiropractic and osteopathic manipulation.

MASSAGE THERAPY

Massage therapy can be beneficial during acute migraine attacks by relieving unhealthful patterns of muscle tension and abnormal posture and by reducing the amount of muscle contraction contributing to the mixed headache (the headache that has features of both a migraine and a tension-type headache). What's more, massage has been proven to increase serotonin levels in both the client and massage therapist, making it an excellent stress buster. From my work with patients, there's no question about the correlation between stress and migraine. Reducing stress in your life can reduce the frequency and severity of your migraines.

Most states license massage therapists. Ask your physician for a referral to a qualified practitioner. If she can't recommend one, you might make inquiries at your local health department or a reputable spa or fitness center. A licensed or fully trained massage therapist will be able to detect abnormal patterns of muscle tension and help you achieve relaxation in specific muscle groups. (While they may feel good, informal neck rubs given by a lover or spouse are no substitute for those provided by a trained and experienced professional.)

PHYSICAL THERAPY

Physical therapy, which is administered by a physical therapist who has extensive knowledge of the musculoskeletal system, involves a combination of massage, therapeutic exercise, and the application of cold or heat for the mobilization of joints and tissues. It can be used to improve abnormal posture in patients or to tackle an unhealthful pattern of muscle tension that can contribute to migraines. Those gains can be maintained with appropriate exercise and massage.

Physical therapy—which is generally covered by health insurance, whereas massage therapy is often excluded—can be effective when massage therapy by itself has failed. While physical therapy is often recommended to manage migraine when patients are pregnant and medication usage is limited or curtailed, I believe that it should be more frequently employed by all migraineurs. When I "prescribe" physical therapy, I recommend that my patients go for eight one-hour sessions, twice a week. Often you will hurt after your first couple of treatments, just as you do after exercising muscles that have been out of use for some time. But hang in there; physical therapy can be extremely effective with migraine.

CHIROPRACTIC MANIPULATION

Several studies have shown chiropractic manipulation to be beneficial for the treatment of headaches that originate in the neck. While little study exists on the effectiveness of chiropractic treatment for migraine in particular, we do know there is a positive, demonstrated association with neck pain. Despite the lack of specific scientific study on migraine, nevertheless, many migraineurs swear by chiropractic manipulation for relief of their headaches. Anecdotal evidence suggests that chiropractic manipulation may be able to stop a migraine attack dead in its tracks but is less likely to act preventively to reduce the frequency and severity of subsequent attacks (unless your chiropractor offers a combination of massage and manipulation). However, the obvious problem with relying on chiropractic treatment for migraine is that it may not be possible to schedule an appointment right when a migraine hits, and it's better to be seen earlier rather than later during the attack.

Patty, forty-three, was reluctant to take preventative medications because of the side effects she'd experienced with several. She had significant neck-muscle tension on examination and so was referred to a chiropractor with special expertise in the treatment of headaches. Patty still has headaches, but they now occur just once or twice a month instead of once a week, and they respond well to a compound analgesic.

A reputable chiropractor will perform a thorough examination along with taking X rays of the neck before doing a manipulation. You should know that cases of stroke (though very rare) have been reported after neck manipulation, whether performed by a chiropractor, physical therapist, or some other practitioner. These have most often occurred when the head was hyperextended, or tipped very far back. However, transient side effects from chiropractic treatment—such as nausea, skin redness, temporary soreness, and/or fatigue—are far more common. One study noted that 10 percent of these reactions involved headaches. This, of course, does not occur in everyone, and such side effects generally last only a few hours.

OSTEOPATHIC MANIPULATION

Like chiropractors, osteopathic physicians also manipulate the spine. The primary difference between the two is in training. Chiropractors receive specialized degrees from colleges of chiropractic, which generally require four years of training. Osteopathic physicians are fully licensed doctors who can prescribe medicine and whose medical training is identical to that of other M.D.'s but who receive additional training in osteopathic manipulation, the techniques of which are similar to chiropractic. (Some osteopathic physicians practice general medicine, whereas others specialize in cardiology, psychiatry, or other medical specialties. A few specialize in the musculoskeletal system.)

Osteopathic manipulation—which involves hand-to-body techniques that attempt to reduce muscle spasm and improve function—can also be effective in treating headaches. While there are no long-term, controlled studies demonstrating a reduction in the rate of migraine occurrence due to osteopathic manipulation, many migraineurs swear by this form of treatment.

BIOFEEDBACK

Biofeedback is a process in which you can learn to control such physical conditions in your body as temperature and blood flow through imaging bodily reactions on a computer screen or a specialized oscilloscope. Though no one knows precisely how this process works, it has proven effective at reducing migraine frequency. Biofeedback is performed by various health care practitioners who have received special training; the first couple of treatments generally take about an hour each in the specialist's office.

Biofeedback was initially developed to help people control their skeletal muscles, which are the muscles that attach to bones and joints, allowing them to move their fingers, toes, arms, legs, et cetera. Three types of biofeedback are used to control migraine:

1. *Temporal arterial biofeedback* teaches you to reduce blood flow through the arteries in your scalp, thus decreasing headache severity and duration. This technique is taught in the specialist's office, but patients are taught to practice it on their own after their first few visits.
2. *Thermal biofeedback* is much easier to perform than the former and thus is used more often. The idea is to change the temperature of a body part by altering blood flow to that part. It's practiced by teaching you, for example, to warm your hands to divert blood from your head. Thermal biofeedback is taught in the specialist's office and is eventually done at home, although periodic follow-ups help assure you that you're practicing it correctly.
3. *Electromyographic* (EMG) biofeedback was initially developed to combat tension-type headaches but can be used effectively in the treatment of migraines. EMG biofeedback is typically performed in the specialist's office. Surface EMG electrodes that pick up either body temperature or muscle tension are attached to different parts of your body and carry information to a computer monitor or an oscilloscope for display. The goal is to reduce your body temperature or relax your mus-

cles by viewing your temperature or your muscular activity on the screen; the patient focuses on changing the oscilloscope pattern—a technique that reportedly is easier to learn than warming your hands or changing the blood flow in your temporal arteries.

While biofeedback does not lend itself to scrutiny by double-blind, placebo-controlled methods, studies of its success rate show it to be superior to the placebo response rate in general.

ACUPUNCTURE

Although most people are initially wary of having needles stuck in them, many migraineurs would gladly offer themselves up as human pincushions if only it would banish a migraine. Acupuncture—the ancient Chinese practice of inserting needles into certain key points in the body to relieve pain or combat disease—has gained increasing popularity in the Western world in recent years.

Attempts to understand this Eastern medical practice—which is over three thousand years old and predates the formal scientific study of anatomy and physiology—in terms of standard anatomy and physiology have been largely unsuccessful. A consensus panel at the National Institute of Health did conclude that acupuncture has shown promising results, although it is difficult to study because it's hard to devise a placebo form of sticking patients with needles. Some critics argue that acupuncture response rates are no better than placebo response rates in the treatment of various conditions. Yet reliable studies have shown success rates from acupuncture treatment to be as high as 75 percent—or much higher than the standard 35 percent or so usually seen in placebo studies.

Because acupuncture does seem to help some people who suffer from such chronic conditions as arthritis, infertility, and migraine, many Western scientists have concluded that it may actually stimulate the release of such helpful neuro-transmitters as endorphins and enkephalins (naturally occurring morphinelike substances that block pain) and adrenocorticotropic hormone (or ACTH, which triggers anti-inflammatory activity). Other researchers have proposed serotonin as the active agent in pain relief achieved from acupuncture.

Complications from acupuncture treatment—such as puncturing a blood vessel or nerve—are infrequent but occa-sionally do happen. What's more, pain can occur at the puncture site, and sometimes people feel light-headed or even faint after treatment. Many states license acupunctur-ists under medical and other professional licensing boards, so check your Yellow Pages for licensing information, and ask around for referrals.

BEHAVIORAL THERAPIES

A number of behavioral-therapy strategies can be effective in reducing migraine pain and/or frequency. These work by one of two methods—relaxing your otherwise tense muscles or attacking the psychological factors that may be contributing to your pain.

RELAXATION THERAPY

Progressive relaxation training is frequently employed in the treatment of headache. With this technique, either a thera-pist or an audiotape will walk you through the process of progressively relaxing each major muscle group in your body until you achieve total relaxation. For example, you might be told to first relax your right hand ("Your right hand is getting heavy"), then your left, then your right arm, then your left—until you're completely relaxed.

Unless you count a tape recorder as machinery, the beauty of this technique is that it involves none. In-person training sessions usually take about thirty minutes and involve first tensing and then relaxing muscle groups, one by one, all over your body. Audiotapes of progressive relaxation technique are commercially available in bookstores and by mail order.

Relaxation therapy can definitely help you relax, and in some women it can cut down on the number and severity of headaches. "I'm a naturally tense person—your typical nervous Nellie," my patient Debbie Jo, thirty-seven, confessed. "But when I learned how to relax myself, it helped immeasurably with my headaches. Now, when I feel a migraine coming on, I turn to relaxation therapy first. It works for me at least half of the time."

HYPNOSIS

Although some migraineurs book sessions with trained hypnotherapists, the type of hypnosis generally used in pain management is self-hypnosis. You can learn this technique from an audiotape or through instruction from a reputable hypnotherapist. The idea is simple: You are in control; you learn to enter a light trance state; you tell yourself not to feel pain. Why this mental state can sometimes block pain remains unclear, physiologically speaking. It may simply cause deep relaxation, or it may bring about neurochemical changes that we have not yet discovered.

But no matter what the physiological explanation, hypnosis can help where nothing else has. I've seen it work magic on patients who had hitherto appeared untreatable. Arden, forty-four, is a case in point. She experienced dreadful headaches, which even injections of Demerol would not relieve. She had tried every medication on the market, but nothing seemed to work for her. But even though she had not responded to an in-office injection of Imitrex earlier that day, she became pain-free during her first hypnotherapy session.

Follow-up counseling also helped Arden. During sessions, she was able to confront the fact of being in an abusive relationship. Once she ended the relationship, her migraines went from being frequent to occasional. "It's amazing how hypnosis has changed my life—restored the quality of my life," Arden told me later. After several sessions with a hypnotist, she learned self-hypnosis. Now, whenever she feels a migraine coming on, she hypnotizes herself.

Though Arden's case may be more dramatic than most, you may want to try hypnotherapy, which could provide you with some relief from your migraines.

MEDITATION AND GUIDED IMAGERY

Some migraineurs report headache relief through meditation, a technique in which you clear your mind of extraneous thoughts and mental clutter in order to concentrate deeply on relaxation. Many meditators develop a specific place—or personal sacred spot—in their minds that represents peacefulness, such as a special mountaintop, a beach, a lake, or some other spot that they "visit" when they meditate.

Jane, forty-five, a migraine sufferer who uses meditation to help control her headaches, almost always "visits" a favorite castle in the Swiss Alps. A framed poster of Jane's Alpine paradise hangs on her bedroom wall. Other meditators simply try to rid their minds of distracting thoughts. As with relaxation therapy, the techniques of meditation and guided imagery can be learned from a therapist or by using one of many popular self-help tapes to guide you along. Any number of books are available on the subject.

"Once I started meditating every morning for forty minutes, I found tremendous relief from my migraines," Mona, a twenty-nine-year-old migraine sufferer, told me.

Guided imagery is similar to meditation, but it specifically involves imagining a pleasant, peaceful, pain-free place and guiding your mind there, away from your corridors of pain. Although neither meditation nor guided imagery has ever had any impact on my own migraines, I have heard too many laudatory accounts from my patients to discount its efficacy. Though we do not fully understand the neurochemistry of such mind-over-body phenomena as meditation, guided imagery, or even hypnosis, these techniques do work for many migraineurs who achieve a degree of pain relief and relaxation by employing them.

PSYCHOTHERAPY

On occasion, psychological stressors may make your migraines worse. In such cases, psychotherapy, which can range from simple counseling to cognitive and behavioral therapy, can help you deal with the problems in your life that may be stirring up your headaches. I've seen many instances among migraineurs in which the pain is psychosomatic; you can work yourself into headaches by suppressing anger and other emotions. If this sounds like it could be your problem, psychotherapy may help you address it by walking you through—and talking you through—the various emotions that may be triggering the onset of migraine.

Some migraineurs also have such frequent headaches that they develop a "fear-of-pain" syndrome. While we all have some aversion to pain, this is an abnormal degree of fear leading to behaviors that are either not helpful or even harmful, such as medication overuse and rebound headache. Psychotherapy can be useful in combating this abnormal fear of pain by helping patients differentiate between emotions.

OTHER REMEDIES TO CONSIDER

Some of the following are old folk remedies; others are trendy new treatments. Any or all may be helpful in relieving your migraine pain.

HEAT OR COLD THERAPY

Most of my patients prefer applying cold rather than heat to help take the edge off their pain. Anna Claire, thirty-six, spoke for many when she reported to me that an ice pack doesn't knock out her headaches, but it does make the wait for her medication to kick in more tolerable.

A variety of commercial ice packs on the market can do the trick, and I've even seen a battery-operated cold cap marketed especially for headache relief. But for most migraineurs, nothing so elaborate is needed. You can easily devise your own ice pack by placing crushed ice or small ice cubes in a resealable plastic bag. Or simply use a small bag of frozen vegetables wrapped in a towel or cloth; frozen peas, since they are round, mold to the shape of your head or neck better than lumpier items. (And after they're defrosted and your head feels better, you can cook them for dinner!)

However, some migraineurs prefer heat to cold. You can put a heating pad or microwaveable gel pack to your head. But bear in mind that heat should not be applied for longer than twenty minutes, and a cloth barrier between the heating pad and your skin should always be used to prevent burning.

Because heat relaxes muscles and increases circulation by dilating surface blood vessels, and cold reduces the swelling brought on by the heat, thus reversing vasodilation of surface blood vessels, some physicians recommend alternating applications of heat and cold. If the muscles in your neck feel tight during your migraine, you might want to consider this treatment.

AROMATHERAPY

Aromatherapy is the practice of inhaling specific odors to achieve physiological or psychological relief from pain, or to help achieve relaxation or sheer olfactory pleasure. Sometimes incense or a scented candle is used; sometimes essential oils are burned over a slow flame or distributed through water in a vaporizer. Research into the psychological, physiological, and therapeutic effects of odors is still in its infancy, but thus far, evidence suggests that aromas may have far-reaching ramifications for our health and overall sense of well-being.

But the sad truth is that the sense of smell remains largely unappreciated by most people. In one recent survey, 55 percent of Americans surveyed said it was the one sense they could do without. Yet your sense of taste is far more limited than your sense of smell; your taste buds can only detect sweet, salt, bitter, and sour. All the other aspects of flavor derive from your sense of smell. And scents can evoke powerful emotions as well as trigger memories.

It's well known in retailing circles that odors can affect consumer behavior; museums and stores frequently use scents to attract customers, finding that people linger longer in stores when pleasant scents are present. Peppermint has been shown to reduce anxiety and increase productivity in the workplace. Both peppermint and green apple scents have been proven to help migraineurs feel better. The scent of lavender is also commonly used to prevent headache. (Historically, taking an extract of lavender internally and applying fresh leaves and flowers directly to the forehead have also been used to treat headaches.) And vanilla fragrance tends to be universally soothing.

A forty-one-year-old patient named Wanda told me that once she hung vanilla sachets in various spots around her bedroom, her headaches decreased in frequency. "The soothing smell also helped me sleep better and more soundly," she said.

While many aromatherapists recommend breathing in scents, others advocate a light massage with scented oils for the treatment of migraine. If you'd like to try self-massage, consider lightly rubbing massage oil laced with peppermint extract into your forehead and temples.

LIFESTYLE CHANGES TO THE RESCUE

Migraines can be affected by a number of lifestyle variables, such as whether you get enough sleep and sleep consistent hours, whether you eat balanced meals, whether you eat regularly, and whether you are moderate and steady in your intake of caffeine and alcohol. Smoking and stress should not be discounted as contributing factors in the onset of migraines. (For more information on common migraine triggers, read Chapter 1.) Following are some ideas that you can incorporate into your lifestyle regimen that may help lessen the number and severity of your migraines.

EXERCISE

A crucial lifestyle factor over which you have significant control is the amount of exercise you get. A regular regimen of aerobic exercise such as running, walking, tennis, bicycling, or swimming will boost your overall levels of fitness and wellness and can help you sleep more soundly.

I know several people who exercise *when* they get a migraine. While this may sound like agony, it can bring about relief through the release of endorphins into your system. My patient Michelle, thirty-six, jogs at the onset of her migraines and obtains relief more often than not. If you've never tried it, I'd recommend a low-impact aerobic activity, such as swimming or walking, over something jarring like jogging or racquetball, during the throes of an attack. I've also heard yoga and Tai Chi advocated for migraine relief. "I'm in a deeply relaxed state after practicing yoga," one of my patients said, "which makes my pain go away."

SEX: THE GREAT HEALER

Just as exercise can help combat the pain of migraine, sexual activity that climaxes in orgasm can also stimulate the release of pain-reducing endorphins in your brain. Just as with exercise, you may not feel like having sex when you're in the throes of a migraine attack, but some of my patients heartily recommend it.

Said Judi, a longtime migraineur, "I have found sexual

arousal to be a decent painkiller. When I have a miserable migraine that's not responding to medications, being sexual with myself can give me a temporary break from pain."

"NATURAL" REMEDIES

Many patients are looking to natural remedies and supplements for migraine relief. The good news is that some of them do work. The bad news is that you need to be skeptical and selective about what you take.

FIVE TIPS FOR TRYING ALTERNATIVE REMEDIES

1. Don't introduce more than one alternative therapy at a time. Do not try an herbal remedy, chiropractic manipulation, and biofeedback all during the same week. If you do and find that you feel better, you'll never know which one worked for you. Plan a time lag of at least two weeks between each new therapy or treatment that you try.

2. Inform your physician before you try an alternative remedy or treatment. If you have tried any of these in the past, make sure your doctor knows about them and whether or not you found them helpful.

3. Don't expect miracles from your natural remedies or therapies. Migraine is a chronic medical problem for which magic-wand–type cures are rare. In most cases, alternative treatments don't completely suppress your migraines, but they may decrease the frequency or severity of your attacks.

4. Don't rely on the medical advice of health food store employees. Do consult your physician or pharmacist, either of whom should have greater knowledge about these remedies.

5. After taking one of these remedies, if you start to feel ill or your migraines seem to be getting worse, stop the remedy or treatment immediately and inform your doctor.

First let me clear up a common misconception that I hear voiced at least once a week from patients: If it's natural, it must be safe. This is not necessarily so. Poison ivy is natural; so is cobra venom. Equating "natural" with "good" or "safe" can lead to serious errors in judgment, avoidable illnesses, and unfortunate herb-drug interactions. Yet many people share this belief. In a survey of women ages eighteen through forty-nine reported in the June 1998 issue of the trade journal *American Druggist*, 42 percent said that "if something is natural, it is good for you." And over half, or 53 percent, of the women surveyed believed herbal/natural remedies were just as good as over-the-counter or prescription medications.

In addition to mistakenly believing all natural remedies to be safe, many patients never tell their physicians that they are taking herbal preparations or natural remedies. A study published in *Archives of Family Medicine* in 1997 revealed that only about 53 percent of those using alternative therapies reported this information to their doctors. Although many people do " 'fess up" to their doctor, too many continue to withhold this information—perhaps fearing their physician's disapproval.

But keeping this information to yourself can be dangerous because no matter how "natural" a remedy is, it can interact with other medications you are currently taking. For example, taking feverfew for migraines at the same time you take a blood thinner such as Coumadin (dicumarol) could result in uncontrollable bleeding.

Tina, thirty-four, a patient with unmanageable daily migraines, came into my office with more than twenty-five herbs and vitamin preparations she was taking in tow. Because these had been recommended by physical therapists and acupuncturists, it had not occurred to her that this daily ingestion of herbs and vitamins might be contributing to— rather than alleviating—her pain. One problem was that each practitioner had recommended something without knowing what else she was taking. While there is no way for me, as her doctor, to know exactly what effects this combination of substances might have been having on Tina, I can assure you that she improved greatly when these substances were discontinued and an appropriate regimen of medication and exercise was started.

Some people fall for the fallacy that "more is better," assuming that if one or two pills work well, then many more will do the job even better. It doesn't work that way: Ten aspirin are *not* ten times better than one. No matter how safe a substance may be, almost anything can be toxic in high-enough doses.

Unfortunately, few controlled studies have been done to assess the safety and efficacy of most herbal supplements. Because of this lack of information, there exists no database on which doctors, pharmacists, or proactive patients can look up drug-herb interactions. Nevertheless, it's imperative that you let your doctor know exactly what remedies you are currently taking or plan to use. As I emphasized in Chapter 2, I recommend that every migraineur do for their physician what Tina did for me. Bring in the bottles and jars of all the medications you're taking—alternative, prescription, and over-the-counter—or at least an exhaustive list.

After cautioning you about the indiscriminate use of natural remedies, let me now report that some of them have been proven by scientific study to work. Even my fellow physicians are impressed with some of the findings on the migraine-averting abilities of several natural substances.

RIBOFLAVIN: THE NATURAL REMEDY OF CHOICE

Several recent studies have demonstrated that high doses of riboflavin (vitamin B-2) can be effective in preventing migraine.

For example, one of the studies, reported in a 1998 issue of *Neurology*, followed migraine sufferers taking 400 milligrams of riboflavin daily and compared them to those on placebo for three months. Of the riboflavin group, 59 per-

CONSUMER ALERT: ARE YOUR SUPPLEMENTS SAFE?

At present, no governmentally sanctioned seal of approval exists for vitamins and herbs that are sold over-the-counter. These natural remedies and herbs do not go through the lengthy and rigorous approval process by the Food and Drug Administration (FDA) that's required for prescription medications. Any safeguards that do exist come from the Federal Trade Commission (FTC), which monitors advertising claims. While truth-in-advertising regulations should prevent outlandish claims of effectiveness, it's unfortunate that these over-the-counter products are not as closely scrutinized as other medicines.

However, the FDA is considering mandating standardized labeling of over-the-counter pharmaceuticals similar to the nutritional labeling now required on processed foods. If approved, such labeling will be required for herbal nutritional supplements. (Recently, another new labeling requirement—which warns of the dangers of taking these medications if you drink three or more alcoholic drinks a day—was implemented for over-the-counter painkillers.)

Presently classified as dietary supplements, herbs, vitamins, amino acids, enzymes, and minerals are regulated under the Dietary Supplement Health and Education Act of 1994, which allows retailers to sell natural remedies or "botanicals" and provide some information on how they might benefit consumers. No proof of safety is required, nor are these products subject to purity standards, which would assure that uniform amounts of the active ingredients of the herb are contained in each tablet. As it stands now, a supplement may be marketed unless the governmental regulatory agencies can prove the product is *not* safe.

When you do buy a dietary supplement, try to stick with a nationally known brand made by a company that is likely to have more quality controls in place and more to lose if a controversy erupts over one of its products.

cent improved by at least 50 percent, while only 15 percent of the placebo group showed that much gain. On average, the patients who improved enjoyed an impressive *68 percent* reduction in the severity of their migraines. (A few of the study participants experienced minor adverse effects, such as diarrhea or excessive urination, which suggests some caution with high doses.)

However, the upside of riboflavin is so strong that I am currently recommending it to my patients as the natural remedy of choice for migraine prevention. It has two noteworthy pluses: It's well-tolerated by most people, and it's inexpensive. But because the usual dose of riboflavin is 25 milligrams and it's not currently commercially available in strengths of 200 or 400 milligrams, you'll need to have higher doses specially made up by a compounding pharmacy. I'm convinced that once this remedy becomes more widely known and accepted, it will be only a matter of time before manufacturers bring riboflavin to market in higher doses. As always, consult your physician before taking riboflavin in doses higher than 100 milligrams daily. And bear in mind that most migraineurs who have tried riboflavin therapy report that it takes two or three months before they see a reduction in migraine frequency and severity.

THE MAGNESIUM QUESTION

Could migraineurs have a lower concentration of magnesium in their bodies than nonmigraineurs? Some researchers think so, and some studies have indicated magnesium supplementation may work with some migraineurs in preventing migraine. It has been theorized that magnesium may affect serotonin levels, altering the release of substance P (a neurotransmitter related to pain) and influencing cells responsible for transmitting pain throughout the nervous system.

However, to date, studies on the effectiveness of magnesium supplements in preventing migraine have presented mixed results, with some showing little or no benefit and others showing different degrees of benefit from various forms of magnesium.

We do know that some migraine sufferers have decreased magnesium levels during a migraine. Some studies also suggest that magnesium levels between headaches may be somewhat lower for migraineurs than for nonmigraineurs. They may not be clinically "deficient" in the classic sense of a vitamin or mineral deficiency, but this subclinically lower level of magnesium could affect brain-magnesium levels and lower the threshold for migraines to occur.

You won't know whether magnesium supplementation will help you unless you try it. If you're interested in doing so, first check with your physician. If I'm treating a patient who is perimenopausal, I generally recommend that she take an over-the-counter calcium/magnesium supplement for a couple of months and see if she shows signs of improvement. Because women need the calcium anyway and the magnesium can't hurt, this is a fairly risk-free avenue. But I might add that I've never seen dramatic results from magnesium supplementation.

FEVERFEW

Feverfew is a plant in the chrysanthemum family that was used in ancient Greece and medieval Europe both to treat headache treatment and to reduce fever. Thanks to the growing popularity of herbal cures and so-called natural treatments, it has enjoyed a recent revival as a migraine preventative. Feverfew grows wild along roadsides and in fields and looks like chamomile; in fact, one of its names is wild chamomile.

Studies of feverfew show it does reduce migraine in about 40 percent of the people who try it. Neurologist Alexander Mauskop, M.D., of the State University of New York Health Science Center in Brooklyn, speculated during his presentation "Alternative Strategies in the Treatment of Migraines" at the June 1998 meeting of the American Association for the Study of Headache that when feverfew works, it's because it's high in magnesium.

The chemical ingredients of feverfew have been isolated by researchers. Feverfew is known to inhibit prostaglandins (circulating substances that cause uterine contractions, resulting in menstrual cramps), which is something aspirin also does, but feverfew does it in a different way. Feverfew also inhibits the release of the neurochemical serotonin from platelets, which is one of the chemical events that occurs in the genesis of a migraine.

Like most other remedies, feverfew has side effects. The most common is mouth ulcers. Lip swelling, loss of taste, and dermatitis have also been reported. Feverfew users who've taken the herb for several years and then stopped abruptly (or switched to a placebo during a study) are known to experience rebound migraine headaches, anxiety, and poor sleep patterns.

Feverfew is not recommended during pregnancy or when breast feeding because its safety has not been established under those conditions. What's more, there are as yet no long-term studies to show the safety (or dangers) of taking feverfew over the years for all migraineurs.

GINGER

Some supporters swear by ginger—a tropical, aromatic, Asiatic plant whose rootstock is widely used as a spice, in perfume, and in medicine—as both an effective migraine treatment as well as an antinausea agent. One study showed ginger to be superior to dimenhydrinate (Dramamine) or a placebo in the prevention of motion sickness, but I am aware of no studies that demonstrate the efficacy of the root in the treatment of migraine. Supplemental use in pregnancy appears safe according to available data, and no adverse effects have been described.

MELATONIN

Melatonin—a hormone that is produced naturally in the pineal gland and dissipates as we grow older—has been proposed as a migraine treatment by some because of its interaction with serotonin. Melatonin may prove to be important in the treatment of migraine, but studies are still in their infancy.

One study showed improvement when melatonin tablets were given with a form of tension-type headache associated with a sleep disorder known as delayed sleep-phase syndrome. Another study, reported in *The Lancet*, revealed melatonin to be effective in preventing jet-lag symptoms. As I mentioned earlier in the book, I've long suffered from migraines after West-to-East Coast travel when crossing time zones. But when I recently traveled to Europe on a transcontinental flight, I took 5 milligrams of melatonin and—much to my delight—found that my jet lag was gone within twenty-four hours and that I suffered no migraines whatsoever! However, because no long-term studies have been conducted, I'm reluctant to take melatonin on a regular basis.

To date, melatonin has been more extensively studied in connection with sleep disorders than with migraine. Although research in this field, while promising, is far from definitive, we do know that melatonin interacts with multiple hormones and neurotransmitters and can alter one's biorhythms. But much more needs to be determined in this extremely complex field before we migraine doctors will be ready to make definitive recommendations.

CHAPTER
9

※

Managing Your Migraines at Work and at Home

Now that you know almost everything about migraines, you're doubtless hankering for some common-sense solutions for dealing with the problem in your everyday life. In this chapter I'll discuss your migraines in the context of the workplace, giving you ideas about how to deal with skeptical coworkers and hard-driving bosses and answering the question of whether migraine is considered a disability under the law. Then I'll turn my attention to more personal issues of coping inside the family, giving you suggestions about how to keep your marriage or relationship alive and how to remain an effective parent while battling migraines.

MIGRAINES AT WORK

Working women who experience recurring migraines often find it difficult to manage headache pain and a demanding job at the same time. Though we do know that almost half of all migraine attacks occur in the morning between the hours of four and nine o'clock—meaning that they're more likely to hit you at home than at work—it's not always possible to pinpoint when one will occur. When one does rear its ugly head at work, an attack could knock you off your feet, derailing a critical presentation or causing you to miss an important deadline or complete some essential task.

Amy, thirty-one, a polished and popular news broadcaster, lived in constant fear that she might experience a migraine while on air. One evening—during a live broadcast of the evening news—it happened. Amy's head began throbbing violently, making it hard for her to read the TelePrompTer and deliver a smooth narration. Even worse, she became nauseated and found herself rushing back and forth to the bathroom during commercial breaks to throw up. Her only blessing was that she didn't vomit on camera. She explained away her problem to her producer as "food poisoning." But after it happened once, Amy decided to change careers.

If you, like Amy, find your migraines causing you anxiety at work, you're not alone. In a study conducted by Opinion Research Corp. for Glaxo Wellcome, nearly half, or 48 percent, of migraineurs surveyed said that their headaches significantly impacted their job performance. Over one-fifth, or 21 percent, said that migraines prevented them from achieving their full work potential. And a huge majority—82 percent—said that their headaches hindered their ability to work at the expected pace.

The right medication, exercise, and lifestyle regimen should help to control your migraines, but what other steps can you take to mitigate your on-the-work woes?

SHOULD YOU TELL YOUR BOSS?

Some women with migraines fear job evaluations, promotions, and their entire careers will be negatively affected if they bring their migraines out into the open. Like Amy, they often make up phony excuses like back pain, arthritis, food poisoning, and even menstrual cramps to hide their condition. In the minds of many migraineurs and nonmigraineurs alike, there remains a stigma about getting migraines, as if these beastly headaches were somehow imaginary, psychosomatic, or mere bids for attention. Contributing to this perception, many migraineurs lament that they don't *look* sick and halfway wish they had scabs, scars, or bandages—any kind of physical marker—that would validate their suffering. Still other migraineurs are overly stoic and often try to "tough out" their headaches, believing this migraine won't be so bad, only to realize later that they're in the midst of a full-blown migraine and they need relief fast. While I don't dispute the notion that some bosses may be unsympathetic and may even behave unreasonably when first approached with the news that you're susceptible to migraines and may be forced to take some "downtime" on the job, I believe an exaggerated fear can cause far more problems than revealing your "secret" will.

Unless you get migraine only once in a blue moon, my best recommendation is to bring the problem out into the open. This way you aren't covering up "mysterious" absences and sudden shifts in mood. Consider the downside: If your boss doesn't know about your migraines, when your performance appears to be suffering, she may jump to false conclusions, suspecting substance abuse, personal problems, or a waning interest in your work. This is especially true if she's had no previous experience with migraine.

What's more, you should broach the subject before your supervisor finds out some other way. "Can you imagine what your boss might think if she walked into the bathroom and saw you shooting up?" asked thirty-seven-year-old Deanna rhetorically. "Even if it was only Imitrex?" Deanna, who has dealt with migraines at work her entire adult life, has made it a "personal policy" to clue in her bosses about her periodic migraines while telling them that her injectable medication keeps it under control. She also presents them with a hand-out on Imitrex, as well as a general-information pamphlet on migraine from her doctor's office.

The best way to win your boss into your corner is to make an appointment to discuss the situation when you both have some free time. Invite her to breakfast or lunch, and make it a point to pick up the tab. Avoid discussing the subject when you're in the middle of a migraine, so you can talk about it coherently and dispassionately. And never bring up the subject when you're standing around shooting the breeze with a bunch of coworkers who might throw their uninformed two cents' worth into the discussion.

When Linda, thirty-six, finally screwed up the courage to tell her boss and coworkers about her migraines, she felt like she was "coming out of the closet." But rather than being met with scorn and derision, Linda was amazed at the supportive response she received.

Likewise, Greta, forty-two, a teacher who had to tell the principal about her migraines because they were starting to occur more frequently at school, found him to be "very understanding." Greta was also impressed with—and touched by—the response of the office staff. "One of the secretaries volunteered to learn how to give shots, in case I was too sick to inject myself."

THE NEGATIVE BOSS

But what if you come up against an unsympathetic boss who simply doesn't "get it"? If he encounters you in the throes of a migraine, he may suggest you take a few aspirins and "pull yourself together." Or, if you schedule an appointment to tell him about your problem, he may dismiss it out of hand or ask questions that imply you're stressed-out or having problems in your personal life. Such a reaction is hardly far-fetched. Indeed, over one-fifth, or 21 percent, of the women with migraines who responded to a nationwide survey conducted for Glaxo Wellcome said their employers were more sympathetic to men with headaches than to women. What's more, fully 13 percent said that employers saw migraine as "an excuse" to avoid doing their work.

What to do about such cases? Alana, twenty-five, told me that no matter how hard she tried to explain the severity of her problem to her boss, it just didn't work. Not until one

TIPS FOR TELLING YOUR BOSS ABOUT MIGRAINE

1. Don't make a big deal out of your migraines. You don't want to make it seem as if your life revolves around them, nor do you want to make yourself out to be a victim.

2. Bring a pamphlet or printed material on migraine that should clear up any misconceptions your boss might have. You can also give him a copy of this book.

3. Explain briefly what you're doing about the problem; for example, you take medication that usually works, although you may be "down" for an hour or so and may need to take a break during this time. That might entail going to the break room to stretch out on the couch and having your calls held until your medication kicks in.

4. Determine whether there are improvements in your work setup that could eliminate migraine triggers, and what your supervisor can do to help. Have suggestions in mind before you walk through his door. For example, if you face glaring sunlight that triggers your headaches, ask that your workstation be repositioned or blinds be installed. If loud noise disturbs you, point out that you would perform your job more quickly and efficiently if moved away from your noisy office adjacent to the loading dock. Or suggest that sound buffers be installed. Keep in mind that the solution must be within your supervisor's reach.

5. Work to become an empathetic presence in your office. Not only is it good for your soul to help others, but it's practical. This way, when you're in need, you can call in your chips. Toni, thirty-two, says that one reason her coworkers are so supportive about her migraines is that when they are sick or need assistance because of a health or personal problem, she's always the first to pitch in.

"When other people see that you will help out when they're sick, they're more likely to return the favor when you're in need," Toni remarked. Remember, this applies to your boss as well. If she's suffering from a family crisis, volunteer to pick up her lunch or dry cleaning—even if it's not in your job description.

day when Alana was violently vomiting in the bathroom and her boss walked in and became alarmed did she finally comprehend what a burden Alana carried with her migraines. But what if Alana's boss still didn't understand and continued to berate her for "goofing off"?

If you explain your migraine problem clearly to your boss and continue to receive negative feedback, you may wish to take the problem to your boss's supervisor. In a large company, you could notify someone in the human resources department. Though your supervisor may resent your going over her head, if you are getting nowhere with her, perhaps a word from her higher-ups could help.

YOUR SIGNIFICANT OTHERS

While you may resort to seeking legal help to remedy your troubles in the workplace, you can never legislate relationships inside your home. If your migraine disease not only affects how you feel and what you're capable of doing but disrupts the family routine and outside plans, it's apparent that the problem belongs not only to you but to your entire family. However, once you lay a foundation for coping with your migraines and a routine for functioning smoothly as a family unit, everyone should feel better while you're down with an attack.

As with explaining your problem at the workplace, it's often hard to break the ice on the subject of change at home, but the stakes are arguably higher for getting your personal house in order. I've heard of marriages breaking up due to the pressures of migraine, so I always advise patients to jump

MIGRAINE AND THE LAW

THE FAMILY AND MEDICAL LEAVE ACT

If things are going so badly that you worry you'll get laid off because of your frequent migraine absences, you may wish to look up your rights under the Family and Medical Leave Act (FMLA). Of course, the best course of action is to be sure you are on the most effective medication regimen possible. Since this may require some trial and error with various medications, the FMLA can help to buy you and your doctor some time until your migraines are under control.

The Family and Medical Leave Act, enacted in 1993, provides for up to twelve weeks of unpaid leave if you've worked 1,250 hours or more (about seven and a half months of full-time employment) for a company with more than fifty employees. This leave may be taken for your own health or for the medical problems of a child or family member who needs assistance. If you wish to invoke the provisions of this act, you must first inform your boss that the reason for your absences is your migraines.

In one case, an employee was laid off for many absences. She did not tell her boss until *after* the layoff that her problem was migraines. Because she had given no one this crucial bit of information while she was still employed, the courts held that the FMLA could not be applied in her situation. However, had she told them that it was migraine, she would have been protected by FMLA because migraine is included in the FMLA section of the law as a "serious condition."

This does not mean you need to take twelve weeks of unpaid leave all at once. It means that you have the option of taking unpaid leave when you've used up all your paid sick leave. The FMLA also provides for leave taken sporadically—several hours here and several hours there—or "intermittently or on a reduced leave schedule for certain conditions." One of these conditions is a "chronic health problem" for which you may need leave for periods ranging from an hour or more to several weeks.

Several lawsuits have been filed by people who were fired from their jobs for absences although they had told their bosses they had a problem with migraines. The employers tried unsuccessfully to have their cases thrown out, alleging that migraine was not a "serious health condition."

While circumstances may compel you to resort to a lawsuit, this has major disadvantages. Litigation is expensive and usually highly stressful. And even if you do win, you'll have to face the animosity of your employer (and possibly your coworkers) when you do return to work. Whenever possible, I recommend you focus your energy on working with your physician to achieve better control of your migraines and taking proactive steps in the workplace to enhance your situation there. For further information about your rights under the FMLA, call the Department of Labor's toll-free number at (800) 959-FMLA.

THE AMERICANS WITH DISABILITIES ACT

Another law that may help women with migraines is the Americans with Disabilities Act (ADA), passed in 1990. Other federal laws ensure that you can't be fired or demoted because of your race, gender, or religion. Similarly, the ADA says people with disabilities can't be terminated because of their disability. If your boss doesn't understand the severity of migraines and decides to demote or fire you because of your headaches, you can complain that you have been discriminated against on these grounds.

Though I dislike equating migraine with "disability," because it is a treatable condition, if you're one of the few who have "tried everything" and still can't shake your severe migraine problem, the ADA may apply to you. As with the FMLA, you must tell your boss about the migraine problem before invoking provisions of the ADA. For more information about the ADA, call (800) 514-0301.

When investigating your rights, check out your state laws, as some are broader than FMLA or the ADA.

in and work on the problem before it wreaks major havoc in their lives.

"My marriage ended because of my migraines," Marion, forty-eight, said emphatically. "My husband couldn't stand being with someone who was sick so much of the time. I missed my son's school plays and parent-teacher meetings and had to cancel any number of vacations and weekend outings we'd planned because I had a migraine on the day of travel."

In fact, Marion could never really commit to an appointment or date because so often sudden migraine attacks forced her to cancel. "I can't drive long distances because if I get a migraine I might end up stranded somewhere. I usually spend two days a week, every week, in the dark, in severe pain." In short, Marion admitted that her life is "centered around" her migraines. And though her husband, Mike, suffered with her for years, finally he reached the breaking point and left the marriage.

Although Marion's case is extreme, many migraineurs believe that their condition strains their marriages. A 1998 study of the impact of migraine on the family reported that 25 percent of those surveyed thought their migraines negatively affected their marriages. And in fully 5 percent of the cases, they believed that their migraines led to their separation or divorce.

What's more, one survey that included questions about sexuality among migraineurs and their spouses revealed that 24 percent of the migraineurs and 23 percent of their spouses answered "yes" when asked if migraines had affected the quality and frequency of their sexual relationship. Nearly one in three migraineurs said that migraines affected their "overall relationship" with their significant other.

But the good news is that while your migraines may affect your relationship—and even the quality of your sex life—the problems don't invariably lead to divorce. Claudia, fifty-three, frequently accompanied her husband, Thom, on business trips where he relied on her to help entertain his clients.

But traveling often brought on her migraines, making her hole up in their hotel room. For several years, Thom believed Claudia was avoiding client meetings and trying to sabotage his career. But with good medication management for Claudia combined with joint marital counseling, they are now working to rebuild their once shaky relationship.

What Your Partner Needs to Know

If your spouse or partner doesn't experience migraines (and the odds are he doesn't), it may be hard for him to comprehend the true extent of your suffering. Though he can't help but notice your weak voice, the vomiting, and the other symptoms you may be experiencing, it may be difficult to comprehend how any "headache" could be this bad.

But even if he does understand what you're going through, he may still resent being burdened with extra duties, such as representing the family at weddings, funerals, school meetings, and plays, and having to cancel dinner parties at the last minute because you're down. Besides seeking treatment, what else can you do to help your partner empathize and understand?

YOU AND THE KIDS

Most mothers with migraines worry a great deal about the impact their illness is having on their children. You fear upsetting and disappointing your kids, and in fact, sometimes you do both. You won't be able to make Tiffany's dance recital or Justin's hockey game because of a migraine. But as long as you explain the reason you have to stay home and as long as you make yourself go whenever you are feeling well, try not to burden yourself with guilt.

You may take comfort in knowing you're not alone. According to a 1995 survey by Opinion Research Corporation, the majority of mothers with migraines believe that their children are adversely affected by their illness. Not only were these mothers concerned about what their children

SIX TIPS FOR BETTER RELATIONSHIPS

1. Learn all you can about migraine in general and your own migraine patterns in particular, then share this information with your partner. Ask him to read pamphlets you've obtained from your doctor or support group. Better yet, ask him to read this book.

2. If there's a migraine support group in your community, sign up. A recent survey revealed that a majority of migraine sufferers (73 percent) felt better after discussing the problem with fellow migraineurs. Whenever possible, invite your significant other to the support group. You may find enormous relief (to say nothing about useful information) from talking with others who experience the same kind of problems that you and your mate are going through. Ask others in the group how they've helped their partners understand the migraine problem and how it affects them. Add your own insights to the pot.

3. Reciprocity helps. As I advised you with coworkers, it's a good idea to be available and ready to pitch in at home when you do not have migraines. Be responsive and understanding when your partner has a medical or work problem. Offer to go the extra mile to help him out when he's under stress.

4. Become a good listener. Good listening means you should avoid getting angry or irritated if your partner expresses frustration or other negative emotions about your migraines. Think back on when your partner was sick and the bulk of the family workload fell on your shoulders. You may have also felt resentment and aggravation. But you realized that it wasn't his fault. This is the position your migraines put him in.

5. While you may freely spend hours helping your child with a school project or perfecting a report for work, you may be stingy about giving yourself a break. Yet we all need unstructured, leisure time to help restore ourselves. Denying

yourself time for mental replenishment increases your stress level, raising the risk of developing a migraine.

6. Don't expect your partner to be saintly. And never assume that you should be perfect yourself. When you're at the top of your game, tell your partner what you'll need from him during an attack. Listen to what he says he's willing to do. Remember, most men are not intuitive about reading body language. And they don't read minds at all.

HIGH-TECH MIGRAINE SUPPORT

Support groups for migraineurs are sprouting up all over the Internet. For example, alt.support.headaches.migraine is a popular group on the World Wide Web. "I am a member of a community of people over the Internet who have experiences similar to mine, and it's very helpful, psychologically," said Suzanne, forty-five, whose migraines started at age thirty. "The support and information that I get is really helpful in managing my migraines." A headache support group is available on CompuServe, and America Online's health forum includes a migraine section.

One caveat, however: Do not assume that everything you read on the Internet or any online service is accurate or up-to-date. While some of the numerous Web sites covering the topic of migraine are managed by professionals, many have been started by individuals with migraine who may not have medical expertise. Be cautious about any medical advice offered by a nonphysician.

might be missing when Mom's sick, but about two-thirds also feared that their children might inherit the illness. (And they may—especially their daughters.)

The survey further revealed that mothers believed that the repercussions of their migraines were significant and that their children had to make special considerations for them, in short, to not act like children. Of the women surveyed, 85 percent believed that their children were forced to refrain from loud activities when they were suffering from migraine; 64 percent believed their children refrained from asking them for their help with homework or personal problems when they were down with migraine.

Helping Your Child to Cope

It can be scary for a child to see his usually competent mother in pain and struggling because of a migraine. It can also inadvertently put the child in the parental role—an unfortunate break in the natural order of things.

Pediatric psychologists and child-development specialists maintain that parents can help their children learn general coping strategies by working toward consistency whenever possible. For example, you could arrange to have meals served at the same time every night, regardless of whether Dad or Mom is the chief cook and bottle washer. The rules should be the same, too. If Mom never lets the dog in a particular room, then Dad shouldn't either. If Mom forbids the TV playing during the dinner hour, Dad should enforce that same rule. Chores that children have when Mom is well should be performed when Mom is sick.

A study on the impact of migraines on the family, reported in the June 1998 issue of *Headache*, revealed some differences between the impact on children under age twelve and that on older children. For example, older children were more "understanding" and "helpful" and less likely to be "hostile" about their parent's migraines than younger children. In the case of younger children, many reacted positively, but 25 percent were "confused" by a parent's migraines; 17 percent were "hostile," and 12 percent were "afraid." In the case of older children, just 12 percent were "hostile."

Younger children are less able to understand a condition like migraine and may find it frightening. This is especially true of children who do not yet grasp time concepts and don't fully understand that Mommy will be better "later." When suffering from migraine around your children, use your common sense and consider the following coping strategies.

OVERCOMING LEARNED BEHAVIOR

As you work to set up positive routines in your family for coping with your migraines, think about the way your family functioned while you were growing up. You can do this yourself, in a support group, or by chatting informally with a friend, or while in therapy. Researchers have found that one reason many people with migraine don't obtain proper treatment—and are sometimes too harsh on themselves—is they've learned poor coping habits while growing up. Nearly half of the migraineurs in one study said that they dealt with their headaches the same way their parents had treated their own headaches when they were growing up. Thus, if Mom took to her bed and didn't take any medication, this pattern could have been unconsciously adopted by her daughter, who as an adult now suffers from migraines.

And if you were unfortunate enough to have developed migraine as a child, think back on how you were treated. If you were not taken seriously, work hard to prevent repeating that pattern with any child of yours who suffers from migraine. And work hard to treat yourself as an adult better than you were treated by your parents. Susan, forty-five, says she was yelled at and spanked at some family outings for not participating. But she could *not* take part because the migraines were so bad. "I cried out that my head hurt, but

DO'S AND DON'TS FOR MOMS WITH MIGRAINES

1. Do work toward consistency. The kids should go to bed at the same time whether Mom is sick or well.

2. Parents should be careful to avoid loading down a child with too many responsibilities. The expectation that a child should care for a parent who is sick—even temporarily—can be very disturbing to the child, who herself needs to be parented.

3. Do not have your children retrieve your medication for you when you're ill. While they can find you an ice pack, turn down the lights, and perform other minor tasks, you should take responsibility for your own medication before you get to the "dragging stage."

4. Instead of having your children tiptoe about the house when you're ill, designate one area where they can play at normal sound levels. This might be the basement, the attic, a porch, or a particular room. If no such place exists inside the house, perhaps the backyard could be the spot. It places a strain on children when it's okay to be raucous in the living room on Monday but they must tiptoe around on Tuesday because Mom is down with a headache.

5. Do reassure your child that you don't have a brain tumor or a terminal illness—only a very bad headache. Many children's movies and fairy tales kill off Mom, so it's not surprising if your children fear that you're much sicker than you are. Often children will not express this fear. So bring it up yourself in a matter-of-fact fashion.

6. Do help younger children (age nine and under) understand. One way to get them to express their feelings is to ask them to draw a picture of a migraine. They may draw a hideous monster. Such a picture could indicate empathy with you. You can also use imagery to describe your migraines, such as how you would like to stuff the migraine in a closet, lock it up, and never let it out again.

7. Don't say you want "to die" when you have a migraine. Children can take such statements very literally, and this could stir up their fears.

8. Do tell your children that your migraines aren't their fault. No matter how loud and unruly your children are, they did not *give* you the susceptibility to migraine.

9. Don't ever use your headache problems as an excuse to avoid going to that dreadful fifth-grade play or your cousin's annual Easter egg hunt. Children aren't stupid; they know more than we realize.

10. Do make a plan for what can be done if a child needs help with homework or needs someone to listen to him practice the clarinet. Can your spouse, your sibling, or an elderly neighbor fill in? Make a backup plan ahead of time. Try to avoid dumping all the responsibility on your significant other. The elderly neighbor down the street may be eager for connection to a younger person. Perhaps if you do things for her (such as trimming her hedges every year or including her in your Thanksgiving dinner), she'd be delighted to pitch in.

11. Do plan ahead. Why not cook extra spaghetti sauce or some other dishes that you can freeze ahead? These can be thawed out and used when you are too ill to manage the cooking.

12. If you can afford it, hire a weekly cleaning service. If you can't afford it, take advantage of your well times to get the house in shape, and make a plan for getting necessary tasks done when you're ill.

13. Don't overload teenagers. They're more responsible than your kindergartener, but they're not adults yet and shouldn't give up their social lives for you. Teenagers are more likely to be willing and able to help you, but try to balance out their needs with yours. Remember that adolescents still need plenty of TLC.

no one believed me," she said, still smarting about her cruel treatment decades ago.

While Susan the adult isn't about to beat herself up, she does need to watch her tendency to be overly stoic. At the same time, it's important not to be too critical of your family when reviewing the past. Give your family members the benefit of the doubt, realizing that they did what they thought was best, whether it involved over-the-counter analgesics, home remedies, or simply putting up with the headache until it was over. If forgiveness is in order, take the first step. And bear in mind that we now know a lot more about migraines than we knew ten or twenty years ago, and our knowledge grows every year. Most of the medications and treatments that we have today were not available to your parents or grandparents years ago.

If you find yourself perpetuating inefficient, old patterns of noncoping that your parents practiced or have developed your own brand of stoicism and self-sacrificial suffering, work on yourself and with your family to break these negative patterns. Be proactive and take solid steps for change.

TELL YOUR FAMILY WHAT YOU NEED DURING MIGRAINES

The best way to be proactive and take solid steps for change inside your family is to express clearly what you need when you're down with a migraine attack. Call a family meeting so that everyone will be on the same page before one strikes. For instance, do you basically need to be left alone? Or do you need Hilda and Russell to rally around, bringing you an ice pack and tending to chores you are unable to do? Is it best if they leave the house for an hour or two?

Sandi, twenty-nine, has put out the word to her children that she has "zero tolerance" for any noise whatsoever during a migraine. "I tell them, no singing, no whistling or radio and that I need to lie down in a dark room until the medicine starts to work."

Karen, forty, a longtime migraineur, said she occasionally has to go to the emergency room. In fact, Karen's sixteen-year-old son, Nathan, was pressed into this very service in the middle of the night on the same day he received his driver's license. She says Nathan was "thrilled" when he had the chance to drive her to the emergency room at two A.M. And Karen felt so sick that she didn't have a chance to worry about his driving skills. They arrived safely, Karen was treated for her headache, and her very grown-up–feeling son then drove her home.

If Karen depended on Nathan as the only person to drive her to the ER or doctor's office when she was ill, she might be seen as overly dependent on her son. However, considering him a backup when her husband was out of town on a business trip is okay.

The main point is that everyone know your expectations of them in advance of when a migraine hits.

CONSIDER FEELINGS

Family members may experience negative feelings with regard to your migraines. They may feel annoyed or angry because you are sick "again" and cannot take them somewhere or accompany them to a special event. They may feel sad, helpless, or distressed because they don't like to see you in this state. Guilt and confusion are common emotions.

It's good to put these emotions out on the table. Do talk about how people can feel when other family members are sick. Express how you felt when your grandmother broke her hip and you had to wait on her hand and foot. This should open the door for your family expressing what they feel when you're down. Talking about what you feel will help validate their feelings and banish some of their anxiety. If your ten-year-old son is angry because you failed to take him to his skating party, he may also feel guilty about his anger. Talking it through can make you both feel better.

WHEN THERAPY CAN HELP

In some cases, you may find that your frequent (or daily) headaches disrupt family interactions and relationships and, though you've done everything within your power to control the problem, your family is on a downward spiral. If so, you may wish to explore family therapy.

If you decide a family therapist can help, seek out someone who's willing to meet with you and provide some insightful analysis after one or two sessions. In most cases, short-term counseling will be all that's necessary. What you need are practical coping strategies. Family therapy can be provided by psychologists, social workers, psychiatrists, or counselors. In general, the therapists with the most advanced training and experience are the most effective.

YOUR EXTENDED FAMILY

Your parents, siblings and their families, and your in-laws—that is, your extended family—may present an even tougher challenge than your immediate family when it comes to behaving empathetically about your migraines. I've heard clients complain about the tactlessness of their mothers-in-law and their husband's cousins—anyone who has never experienced the pain of migraine.

"I suppose you'll get one of your headaches," is what a relative sarcastically told Megan, thirty-four, a migraine patient of mine, when describing a family reunion that was being planned. Megan gritted her teeth and said nothing. It would have been better if she had answered her back, saying something like: "I do have a problem with migraines, like millions of other women, and my doctor is working with me on controlling them. I certainly hope I can make it to the family reunion. But, yes, it's always possible that I might get sick and be unable to attend."

And it's true: No matter how strong your intentions, sometimes the migraine moves in and messes up your plans.

Holidays and family gatherings are especially stressful times for many of us. There are many associated factors that may act as migraine triggers. You may not get enough sleep. Travel may be required to get to the event. You may be exposed to unfamiliar smells, such as cigarette smoke, and strange noises, light patterns, foods, and pets. And merely dealing with problematic family members and issues can in itself add to your stress level.

If you do get a migraine at such a gathering, try to ignore sarcastic remarks. Go to a dark, quiet room and shut the door. Hang a DO NOT DISTURB sign on the door, or put out the word in advance of your retreat. When you're well again, explain what happened and resume your normal plans. If family members continue to verbally abuse you about your migraines, you may wish to limit your contact with them.

MIGRAINES AND YOU

Let's assume you've used the information in this chapter to create more positive and accommodating relationships at work and at home. By taking a proactive stance in your workplace and with members of your immediate and extended families, you've been able to minimize the impact of your migraines. I've already touched on factors from your personal and emotional history that you need to deal with to help you along the way. What else could possibly be holding you back? There remain several salient psychological factors that could contribute to your incidence of migraine. The most important of these is fear.

THE FEAR FACTOR

Fear of migraines can be a prevalent issue for many women who have periodic and acute migraines. A study by Oklahoma physician Hanna Saadah revealed that fear of migraines was a dominant factor in taking analgesics ahead of time, just in case.

Saadah found that in the control group (three headaches per month), the average number of painkillers taken per month was 7. In the "episodic" group, patients with an average of six migraines per month, the average number of analgesics was 22 per month. In the "intractable" group, with an average of twenty-nine migraines per month, the average number of analgesics was a whopping 139.

"I theorize that headache fear reinforces compulsive analgesic overuse and interferes with analgesic withdrawal," concluded Saadah. "Furthermore, the resistance to analgesic withdrawal seems directly proportional to the intensity of fear."

Clearly, at twenty-nine migraines a month and 139 analgesic doses, this intractable group is likely suffering from rebound-headache phenomenon. Their difficulty in withdrawing from medication is due to recurrent rebound headache as well as fear of headache. Fear of migraine, however, is often what creates the problem in the first place. Because of the fear of developing a headache, an analgesic is taken "just in case." This can result in the development of altered pain modulation by the brain, causing rebound headaches.

How do you fight the fear? An effective preventative regimen and an effective plan for treating the migraines that do occur despite prevention is a good start. But if fear is significant and persistent, counseling with someone specializing in pain management may be helpful. Ask your doctor for a recommendation.

And remember, never take painkillers when you don't have a headache. They really won't prevent a migraine from occurring.

DEVELOPING COMPETENCE

By following the advice I offer throughout this book, you can work to gain control over your headaches. The more mastery you achieve over your migraines at work and at home, the more competent you will feel about this and all aspects of your life. Indeed, as you grow with (and despite) your migraines, the better able you will be to deal with the migraines that you do experience, and the more empowered you will be to confront this and other significant problems in your life. Learning to survive—and even thrive—with your migraines may help you shed them entirely someday. And it certainly will help you step forward into your future with a positive outlook.

Epilogue

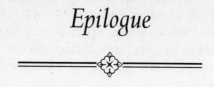

Migraine and the Future

Conscientiously following the steps, suggestions, and ideas offered in this book will help you better manage your migraines and can make an enormous difference in the quality of your life. In fact, this entire book presents the best and most state-of-the-art information available about preventing, coping with, and minimizing these headaches that have been plaguing women (and men) since the beginning of recorded time. Indeed, an ancient Babylonian poet describes migraines as "flashes like lightning," and a misguided Renaissance thinker postulated that migraines were a result of insects crawling inside the brain. Given the rapid pace of medical research, what developments are we likely to see in the treatment of migraine in the future? Will some form of therapy, vaccine, or magic-bullet shot or pill be invented that puts these beastly headaches to rest once and for all?

A BRIGHTER TOMORROW

When you consider just how far we've come in the treatment of migraine in the recent past alone, the future looks bright.

Effective treatment for migraine has only been available in this century, with most methods coming in the latter half. And many new medications, such as the triptans, which work on the serotonin receptors located on the surface blood vessels of the brain, have arrived on the scene as recently as the mid-1990s.

BIOCHEMICAL CAUSES

While we know many of the things that trigger a migraine, we have not yet determined the precise biochemistry in the brain that allows one to develop and take hold. We do know that migraines begin in the part of the brain known as the brainstem, setting off a chain of events, ultimately causing the dilation of the blood vessels on the surface of the brain. The dilation of these meningeal vessels triggers the release of various pain-causing neurotransmitters and stimulates nerve fibers that, in turn, activate pain centers in the brain.

Our present understanding of migraine is that both the brain and blood vessels are involved. This is referred to as trigeminovascular theory. (The trigeminal nerve supplies sensation to the face and to the blood vessels in the brain.) The blood vessels on the surface of the brain each have branches of the trigeminal nerve that connect them to the brainstem, sending messages back and forth. We know that several brain chemicals are involved in these junctions between nerve and blood vessel, which include serotonin, neurokinin, substance P, calcitonin gene-related peptide (CGRP), and GABA (gamma-aminobutyric acid). Each of these chemical interactions within the brain represents a point at which it may be possible to intervene and block the sequence of events that results in a migraine.

GENETICS AND MIGRAINE

When looking at the future of migraine, it is impossible to ignore the genetic factor, which has emerged as a hot topic of research. If we can determine which gene or genes are responsible for the inheritance of the tendency toward migraine, we may be able to accurately predict who is at risk for developing the disease. Although ethically controversial, gene therapy will one day be possible.

THE BIG, BRIGHT PICTURE

As our understanding of the causes and the brain chemistry of migraine expands, I predict that we will move closer and closer to the complete suppression—or even total eradication—of migraine. The next century should prove even more fruitful in bringing results of migraine research and treatment, making the future for migraineurs very bright indeed.

Appendix A
Regional Women's Health Coordinators

This is a listing of the ten regional coordinators for the U.S. Public Health Service Office On Women's Health in the U.S. and its territories. Coordinators convene public meetings, compile information on women's health statistics and resources and promote women's health services and research and education on women's health issues.

Contact the regional coordinator nearest to you to learn about seminars and programs on a variety of women's health and wellness issues.

REGION I: CT, MA, ME, NH, RI, VT
Laurie Robinson, M.T.S.
Women's Health Coordinator
John F. Kennedy Federal Building, Room 2126
Boston, MA 02203
617-565-1071

REGION II: NJ, NY, Puerto Rico, Virgin Islands
Sandra Estepa, M.S.
Women's Health Coordinator
26 Federal Plaza, Room 3835
New York, NY 10278
212-264-4628

REGION III: DC, DE, MD, PA, VA, WV
Rosa F. Myers, A.R.N.P., M.S.N.
Women's Health Coordinator
150 S. Independence Mall West, Suite 436
Philadelphia, PA 19106-3499
215-861-4637

REGION IV: AL, FL, GA, KY, MS, NC, SC, TN
Clara H. Cobb, M.S.N., R.N., C.F.N.P.
Women's Health Coordinator
61 Forsyth Street SW, 5B95
Atlanta, GA 30303-8909
404-562-7904

REGION V: IL, IN, MI, MN, OH, WI
Michelle Hoersch, M.S.
Women's Health Coordinator
105 West Adams, 17th Floor
Chicago, IL 60603
312-353-8122

REGION VI: AR, LA, NM, OK, TX
Shannon Hills, M.P.A.
Women's Health Coordinator
1301 Young Street, Suite 1124
Dallas, TX 75202
214-767-3523

REGION VII: IA, KS, MO, NE
Joyce Twonser, R.N., B.S.N.
Women's Health Coordinator
601 East 12th Street, Room 210
Kansas City, MO 64106
816-426-2829

REGION VIII: CO, MT, ND, SD, UT, WY
Laurie Konsella, M.P.A.
Women's Health Coordinator
1961 Stout Street, Room 498
Denver, CO 80294-3538
303-844-6163, ext. 390

REGION IX: AZ, CA, HI, NV, American Samoa, Guam, Trust Territory of the Pacific Islands

Kay A. Strawder, J.D., M.S.W.
Women's Health Coordinator
50 United Nations Plaza, Room 327
San Francisco, CA 94102
415-437-8119

REGION X: AK, ID, OR, WA

Karen Matsuda, M.N., R.N.
Acting Women's Health Coordinator
2201 Sixth Avenue, M/S RX-29
Seattle, WA 98121
206-615-2501

Appendix B
Other Resources

American Council for Headache Education
19 Mantua Road
Mt. Royal, NJ 08061
1-800-255-ACHE
www.achenet.org

M.A.G.N.U.M., Inc.
113 South Saint Asaph, Suite 300
Alexandria, VA 22314
703-739-9384
703-739-2432 (Fax)
www.migraines.org

National Headache Foundation
428 W. St. James Place, 2nd Floor
Chicago, IL 60614
1-777-388-6394
www.headaches.org

World Headache Alliance
208 Lexington Road
Oakville, Ontario, Canada
L6H 6L6
905-257-6229
905-257-6239 (Fax)
www.w-h-a.org

Bibliography

Abdul Jabbar, M. and A. Ogunniyi. "Sociodemographic factors and primary headache syndromes in a Saudi community." *Neuroepidemiology* 16, no. 1(1997): 48–52.

American Academy of Pediatrics Committee on Drugs. "The Transfer of Drugs and Other Chemicals into Human Milk." *Pediatrics* 93(1994): 137–50.

Baloh, Robert W., M.D. "Neurotology of Migraine." *Headache* 37(November–December 1997): 615–21.

Barrett, Stephen. "Homeopathy: Much Ado About Little or Nothing." *Nutrition Forum* 15(May–June 1998): 17–21.

Bic, Z., et al. "In Search of the Ideal Treatment for Migraine Headache." *Medical Hypotheses* 50(January 1998): 1–7.

Biggs, et al. "Platelet aggregation in patients using feverfew for migraine." *Lancet* 2(1982): 776 Letter.

Bird, Kathleen. "Migraine Sufferers: Protected Class?" *New Jersey Law Journal* 137(May 30, 1994): 1, 33.

Blanchard, E. B., F. Andrasik, T. A. Ahles, et al. "Migraine and tension headaches: a meta-analytic review." *Behavioral Therapy* 11(1980):613–31.

Blau, J. N. "Migraine in Doctors: Work Loss and Consumption of Medication." *The Lancet* 344(December 10, 1994): 1623–24.

Blau, J. N. "The Effect of National Lifestyles." *Cephalgia*, Supplement 21(1998): 23–25.

Breslau, N., and G. C. Davis, "Migraine, physical health and psychiatric disorders: a prospective epidemiologic study of young adults." *Journal of Psychiatric Res* 27 (1993): 211–21.

Brown, A. M., M. Ho, D. R. Thomas, A. A. Parsons. "Comparison of functional effects of frovatriptan (VML 251), sumatriptan, and naratriptan on human recombinant 5-HT$_1$ and 5-HT$_2$ receptors." *Headache* 38(1998): 376.

Chapman, S. L. "A Review and Clinical Perspective on the Use of EMG and Thermal Biofeedback for Chronic Headaches." *Pain* 27(1986): 1–43.

Chen, T. C., and A. Leviton. "Headache recurrence in pregnant women with migraine." *Headache* 34(1994): 107–10.

Clarke, C. E., L. MacMIllan, S. Sondhi, N. E. Wells. "Economic and social impact of migraine." *Quarterly Jounal of Medicine* 89(1996)(1): 77–84.

Collaborative Group on Hormonal Factors in Breast Cancer. "Breast cancer and hormone replacement therapy: collaborative reanalysis of data from 51 epidemiological studies of 52,705 women with breast cancer and 108,411 women without breast cancer." *Lancet* 350(1997): 1047–59.

Culler, N., G.R. Mushet, R. Davis, B. Clements, L. Whitcher, "Oral sumatriptan for the acute treatment of migraine: evalution of three dosage strengths." *Neurology* 45, no. 7(1995): S55-S59.

Dartigues, J. F., et al. "Comparative View of the Socioeconomic Impact of Migraine Versus Low Back Pain." *Cephalalgia* 18, no. 21(February 1998): 26–29.

De Matteis, G., et al. "Geomagnetic Activity, Humidity, Temperature and Headache: Is There Any Correlation?" *Headache* 34(January 1994) 34: 41–43.

Devlen, J. "Anxiety and depression in Migraine." *Journal of R Soc Medicine* 87, no. 6(1994): 338–41.

Drummond, Peter D. "Photophobia and Autonomic Responses to Facial Pain in Migraine." *Brain: A Journal of Neurology* 120(October 1997): 1857–64.

Edmeads, John G., M.D., et al. "Strategies for Diagnosing and Managing Medication-Induced Headache." *Canadian Family Physician* 43(July 1997): 1240–54.

Edmeads, John, M.D. "Headaches in Older People." *Postgraduate Medicine* 101(May 1997): 91–100.

Eisenberg, David M., M.D. "Advising Patients Who Seek Alternative Medical Therapies." *Annals of Internal Medicine* 127(July 1997): 61–69.

Elder, Nancy C., M.D., et al. "Use of Alternative Health Care by Family Practice Patients." *Archives of Family Medicine* 6(March–April 1997): 181–84.

Essink-Bot, Marie-Louise, M.D., et al. "The Impact of Migraine on Health Status." *Headache* 35(April 1995): 200–206.

Facchinetti, F., et al. "The Efficacy and safety of subcutaneous sumatriptan in the acute treatment of menstrual migraine." *Obstetrics Gynecology* 86(1995): 911–16.

Ferrari, Michael D. "Migraine." *The Lancet* 351(April 4, 1998): 1043–51.

Fischer-Rasmussen, W., et al. "Ginger treatment of hyperemesis gravidarum." *European Journal of Obstetrics and Gynecological Reproductive Biology* 38, no. 1(1991): 19.

Forsyth, P. A., and J. B. Posner. "Headaches in patients with brain tumors: a study of 111 patients." *Annals of Neurology* 32(1992): 289

Gallai, V., P. Sarchielli, P. Morucci, G. Abbritti. "Red Blood Cell Magnesium Levels in Migraine Patients." *Cephalalgia* 13(February 1993): 74–81.

Gasbarrini, Antonio, M.D., et al. "Beneficial Effects of Helicobacter pylori Eradication on Migraine." *Hepato-Gastroenterology* 45(1998): 765–70.

Genzen, Jonathan R. "The Internet and Migraine: Headache Resources for Patients and Physicians." *Headache* (April 1998)38: 312–14.

Goldstein, J. "Update: What's New in Headache Drugs?" *Headache Quarterly* Supplement (1997): 28–32.

Goldstein, J., K. Britch, S. Silberstein. "Ganaxolone: New non-triptan shows utility for acute migraine." *Cephalalgia* 18(1998): 393.

Gotoh, F., T. Kandra, F. Sakai, M. Yamamoto, T. Takeoka. "Serum dopamine-beta-hydroxylase activity in migraine." *Archives of Neurology* 33(1976): 656–57.

Grady, D., T. Gebretsadik, K. Kerlikowske, V. Ernster, D. Petitti. "Hormone replacement therapy and endometrial cancer risk: a meta-analysis." *Obstetrics and Gynecology* 85(1995): 304–13.

Grady, D., S. B. Hulley, C. Furberg. "Venous thromboembolic events associated with hormone replacement therapy." *JAMA* 278(1997): 477.

Grady, D., S. M. Rubin, D. B. Petitti, C. S. Fox, D. Black, B. Ettinger et al. "Hormone Therapy to Prevent Disease and Prolong Life in Postmenopausal Women." *Annals of Internal Medicine* 117 (1992): 1016–37.

Granella, F., et al. "Migraine without aura and reproductive life events: A clinical epidemiological study in 1300 women." *Headache* 33(1993): 385–89.

Gruber, Amanda J., et al. "The Management of Treatment-Resistant Depression in Disorders on the Interface of Psychiatry and Medicine: Fibromyalgia, Chronic Fatigue Syndrome, Migraine, Irritable Bowel Syndrome, Atypical Facial Pain, and Premenstrual Dysphoric Disorder." *The Psychiatric Clinics of North America* 19(June 1996): 351–69.

Hay, K. M., M. J. Mortimer, D. C. Barker, L. M. Debney, P. A. Good, "1044 Women with Migraine: The Effect of Environmental Stimuli." *Headache* 34(1994): 166–68.

Hebel, Steven K., Ed. "The Lawrence Review of Natural Products Monograph System." *Facts and Comparisons* (1996): St. Louis, MO.

Helm, J. E., C. Lokken, T. C. Myers. "Migraine and Stress: A Daily Examination of Temporal Relationships in Women Migraineurs." *Headache* 37(1997): 553–58.

Heptinstall, S., et al. "Extracts of feverfew may inhibit platelet behaviour via neutralization of sulphydryl groups." *J Pharm Pharmacol* 39 (1987): 459.

Ho, K. H., B. K. Ong, S. C. Lee. "Headache and Self-assessed Depression Scores in Singapore University Undergraduates," Headache 37, no. 1(1997):26–30.

Hobbs, C., "The Modern Rediscovery of Feverfew," *National Headache Foundation Newsletter* (Winter 1990): 10–11.

Holm, Jeffrey E., Ph.D., et al. "Migraine and Stress: A Daily Examination of Temporal Relationships in Women Migraineurs," *Headache* 37(1997): 553–58.

Honkasalo, M. L., J. Kaprio, K. Heikkilä, M. Sillanpää, M. Koskenvuo. "A population-based survey of headache and migraine in 22,809 adults." *Headache* 33(1993): 403–12.

Isler, H. "Background to the Headaches: Historical Background." In: J. Olesen, P. Tfelt-Hansen, K. M. A. Welch, eds., *The Headaches* (New York: Raven Press, 1993), 1–8.

Johnson, E. S., et al. "Efficacy of Feverfew as Prophylactic Treatment of Migraine." *British Journal of Medicine* 291(1985): 569.

Johnson, Glenn D., M.D. "Medical Management of Migraine-Related Dizziness and Vertigo." *Laryngoscope* 108(January 1998): 1–28.

Kauppila, A., A. Kivel, A. Pakarinen, O. Vakkuri. "Inverse seasonal relationship between melatonin and ovarian activity in humans in a region with a strong seasonal contrast in luminosity." *Journal of Clinical Endocrinology and Metabolism* 65(1987): 823–28.

Kudrow, L. "The Relationship of Headache Frequency to Hormone Use in Migraine." *Headache* 15(1975): 36–49.

Lance, J. W. "Headaches Related to Sexual Activity." *Journal of Neurological Neurosurgery and Psychiatry* 39(1976): 1226–30.

Laya, M. B., E. B. Larson, S. H. Taplin, E. White. "Effect of Estrogen Replacement Therapy on the Specificity and Sensitivity of Screening Mammography," *Journal of National Cancer Inst* 88(1996): 643–69.

Legg, Randall F., et al. "Cost Benefit of Sumatriptan to an Employer." *Journal of Occupational and Environmental Medicine* 39(July 1997): 652–58.

Leviton, A., B. Malvea, J. R. Graham. "Vascular Diseases, Mortality, and Migraine in the Parents of Migraine Patients." *Neurology* 24(1974): 669–72.

Lichten, E. M., J. B. Lichten, A. J. Whitty, D. Pieper. "The use of leuprolide acetate in the diagnosis and treatment of menstrual migraine: the role of artificially induced menopause." *Headache Quarterly* 6, no. 4(1995):313–17.

Lichten, E. M., J. B. Lichten, A. J. Whitty, D. Pieper. "The Confirmation of a Biochemical Marker for Women's Migraine: The Depo-Estradiol Challenge Test." *Headache* 36(1994): 367–70.

Limouzin-Lamothe, M. A., N. Mairon, C. R. B. Joyce, M. De Gal. "Quality of Life After the Menopause: Influence of Hormonal Replacement Therapy." *American Journal of Obstetrics and Gynecology* 170 (1994): 618–24.

Lipton, R. B., W. F. Stewart."Migraine Epidemiology: Perspectives for the Primary Care Provider." *Headache Quartery* (1997): S15–S21.

Lipton, R. B., W. F. Stewart, D. Simon. "Medical Consultation for Migraine: Results From the American Migraine Study." *Headache* 38(1998): 87–96.

Lipton, R. B., W. F. Stewart, M. von Korff. "Burden of Migraine: Societal Costs and Therapeutic Opportunities," *Neurology* 48, no. 3 (1997): S4–S9.

Lipton, Richard B., M.D., and W. F. Stewart, Ph.D. MPH. "Prevalence and Impact of Migraine." *Neurologic Clinics* 15 (February 1997): 1–11.

Lipton, Richard B., and W. F. Stewart, Ph.D. MPH. "Migraine Headaches: Epidemiology and Comorbidity." *Clinical Neuroscience* 5(1998): 2–9.

MacArthur, C., M. Lewis, E. G. Know. "Health After Children." *British Journal of Obstetrics and Gynecology* 98(1991): 1193–1204.

MacGregor, E. A. "Hormone-Related Headaches." *Cephalalgia* 18(1998): 228–29.

MacGregor, E. A., H. Chia, R. C. Vohrah, et al. "Migraine and Menstruation: A Pilot Study." *Cephalalgia* 10, no. 6(1990): 305–10.

Maggioni, F., C. Alessi, T. Maggino, G. Zanchin. "Headache During Pregnancy." *Cephalalgia* 17, no. 7(1997): 765–69.

Magos, A. L., M. Brincat, K. J. Zilkha, J. W. W. Studd. "Serum Dopamine-beta-hydroxylase Activity in Menstrual Migraine." *Journal of Neurological Neurosurgery and Psychiatry* 48(1985): 328–31.

Main, Alan, M. Sc, et al. "Photophobia and Phonophobia in Migraineurs Between Attacks." *Headache* 37(Sept. 1997): 492–95.

Mannix, Lisa K., M.D., et al. "Alcohol, Smoking, and Caffeine Use Among Headache Patients." *Headache* 37(October 1997): 572–76.

Marcus, D. A., L. Scharff, D. Turk, L. M. Gourley. "A Double-blind Provocative Study of Chocolate as a Trigger of Headache." *Cephalalgia* 17, no. 8(1997): 855–62.

Marks, D. A., B. L. Ehrenberg. "Migraine-related seizures in adults with epilepsy, with EEG correlation." *Neurology* 43(1993): 2476–83.

Mauskop, A., B. T. Altura, R. Q. Cracco, B. M. Altura. "Intravenous Magnesium Sulfate Relieves Acute Migraine In Patients With Low Serum Ionized Magnesium Levels." *Neurology* 45, no. 4(1995): A379.

Mauskop, A., B. T. Altura, R. Q. Cracco, B. M. Altura. "Intravenous Magnesium Sulfate Relieves Migraine Attacks in Patients with Low Serum Ionized Magnesium Levels: a Pilot Study." *Clinical Science (Colch)* 89, no. 6(1995): 633–36.

Mauskop, A., B. T. Altura, R. Q. Cracco, B. M. Altura. "Intravenous Magnesium Sulfate Rapidly Alleviates Headaches of Various Types." *Headache* 36(1996): 154–60.

Mauskop, Alexander, and Burton M. Altura. "Role of Magnesium in the Pathogenesis and Treatment of Migraines." *Clinical Neuroscience* 5(January 1998): 24–27.

Mauskop, Alexander, M.D., F.A.A.N., and Marietta Abrams Brill. "The *Headache Alternative: A Neurologist's Guide to Drug-Free Relief*" (New York: Dell Trade Paperback, 1997).

Moskowitz, M.A. "The Neurobiology Of Vascular Head Pain." *Ann-Neurol* 16, no. 2(1984): 157–68.

Mounstephen, A. H., and R. K. Harrison. "A Study of Migrane and Its Effects in a Working Population." *Occupational Medicine* 45(1995): 311–17.

Murialdo, G., Fonzi, S., Costelli, P., Solinas, G. P., Parodi, C., Marabinas, S., Fanciullacci, M., Polleri, A. "Urinary Melatonin Excretion Throughout The Ovarian Cycle In Menstrually Related Migraine." *Cephalalgia* 14, no. 3(1994): 205–9.

Murray, S. C., K. N. Muse. "Effective Treatment of Severe Menstrual Migraine Headaches with Gonadotropin-Releasing Hormone Agonist and "Add-Back" Therapy." *Fertil Steril* 67, no. 2(1997): 390–93.

Mustafa, T., K. C. Srivastava. "Ginger (Zingiber Officinale) in Migraine Headache." *Journal Ethnopharmcol.* 29(1990): 267–73.

Nagtegaal, J. E., M. G. Smits, A. C. Swart, G. A. Kerkhof, Y. G. van der Meer. "Melatonin-Responsive Headache in Delayed Sleep Phase Syndrome: Preliminary Observations." *Headache* 38 (1998): 303–7.

Nattero, G., G. Allais, C. De Lorenzo, et al. "Relevance of Prostaglandins in True Menstrual Migraine." *Headache* 29, no. 4(1989): 233–38.

Neri, I., F. Granella, R. Nappi, G. C. Manzoni, F. Facchinetti, A. R. Genazzani. "Characteristics of Headache at Menopause: A Clinico-Epidemiologic Study." *Maturitas* 17(1993): 31–37.

Newcomb, P. A., and B. E. Storer. "Postmenopausal Hormone Use and Risk of Large-Bowel Cancer." *Journal National Cancer Inst.* 87 (1995): 1067–71.

Newman, L. C., R. B. Lipton, C. L. Lay, S. Solomon. "A Pilot Study of Oral Sumatriptan as Intermittent Prophylaxis of Menstruation-Related Migraine." *Neurology* 51(1998): 307–9.

Newton, K. M., A. Z. LaCroix, B. McKnight, R. H. Knopp, D. S. Siscovick, S. R. Heckbert, et al. "Estrogen Replacement Therapy and Prognosis After First Myocardial Infarction." *American Journal Epidemiol.* 145(1997): 269–77.

Norman, B., D. Panebianco, G. A. Block. for the L–758,298 003 Study Group, West Point, PA, USA. "A Placebo-Controlled, In-Clinic Study to Explore the Preliminary Safety and Efficacy of Intravenous L–758,298 (a Prodrug of the NK$_1$ Receptor Antagonist L–754,030) in the Acute Treatment of Migraine." *Cephalalgia* 18(1998): 407.

O'Dea, J. P. K., and E. H. Davis. "Tamoxifen in the Treatment of Menstrual Migraine." *Neurology* 40, no. 9(1990): 1470.

Oral Sumatriptan and Aspirin Plus Metoclopramide Comparative Study Group. "A Study to Compare Oral Sumatriptan with Oral Aspirin Plus Oral Metoclopramide In The Acute Treatment of Migraine." *European Neurology* 32(1992):177–84.

Ottman, R. O., and R. B. Lipton. "Comorbidity of Migraine and Epilepsy." *Neurology* 44(1994): 2105–10.

Paganini-Hill, A. "Estrogen Replacement Therapy and Stroke." *Progr. Cardiovasc. Dis.* 38(1995): 223–42.

Paiva, T., A. Batista, P. Martins, A. Martins. "The Relationship

Between Headaches and Sleep Disturbances." *Headache* 35, no. 10(1995): 590–96.

Palevitch, D., et al. "Feverfew (Tanacetum parthenium) as a Prophylactic Treatment for Migraine: A Double-Blind Placebo-Controlled Study." *Phytotherapy Research* II(1997): 508–11.

Paulson, G. W., and H. L. Klawans. "Benign Orgasmic Cephalgia." *Headache* 13(1974): 181–87.

Peatfield, M.D. "Relationships Between Food, Wine, and Beer-Precipitated Migrainous Headaches." *Headache* 35(June 1995): 355–57.

Peikert, A., C. Wilimzig, R. Khne-Volland. "Prophylaxis of Migraine with Oral Magnesium: Results from a Prospective, Multi-center, Placebo-controlled and Double-blind Randomized Study." *Cephalalgia* 16, no. 4(April 1996): 257–63.

Peng, A., and W. Greenfield. "A Precise Scientific Explanation of Acupuncture Mechanisms: Are We on the Threshold?" Editorial Review. *Acupunct. Sci. Int. Journal* 1(1990): 28–29.

Peroutka, Stephen J., M.D., Ph.D. "Dopamine and Migraine." *Neurology* 49(September 1997): 650–56.

Petitti, D. B., S. Sidney, J. A. Perlman. "Increased Risk of Cholecystectomy in Users of Supplemental Estrogen." *Gastroenterol.* 94(1988): 91–95.

Pfaffenrath, V., et al. "Magnesium in the Prophylaxis of Migraine—A Double-Blind Placebo-Controlled Study." *Cephalalgia* 16(October 1996): 436–40.

Phebus, L. A., K. W. Johnson, J. M. Zgombick, P. J. Gilbert, K. Vanbelle, V. Mancuso, et al. "Characterization of LY344864 as a Pharmacological Tool to Study $5HT_{1F}$ Receptors—Binding Affinities, Brain Penetration and Activity in the Neurogenic Dural Inflammation Model of Migraine." *Life Science* 61(1997): 2117–26.

Piorecky, J., W. J. Becker, M. S. Rose. "Effect of Chinook Winds on the Probability of Migraine Headache Occurrence." *Headache* 37(March 1997): 153–58.

Porter, M., G. C. Penney, D. Russell, E. Russell, A. Templeton. "A Population Based Survey Of Women's Experience of the Menopause." *British Journal of Obstetrics Gynaecol.* 103(1996): 1025–28.

Pradalier, A., J. M. Launay. "Immunological Aspects of Migraine." *Biomed. Pharmacother.* 50, no. 2(1996): 64–70.

Ramadan, N. M., H. Halvorson, A. Vande-Linde, et al. "Low Brain Magnesium in Migraine." *Headache* 29(1989): 416–19.

Rapoport, A. M., and J. U. Adelman. "Cost of Migraine Management." *American Journal of Managed Care* 4(April 1998): 531–45.

Raps, E. C., J. D. Rogers, S. L. Galette, et al. "The Clinical Spectrum of Unruptured Intracranial Aneurysms." *Arch. Neurol.* 50(1993): 265–68.

Reid, R. L., and S. S. C. Yen. "Premenstrual Syndrome." *American Journal Obstet. Gynecol.* 139(1981): 85–104.

Resnick, S. M., E. J. Metter, A. B. Zonderman. "Estrogen Replacement Therapy and Longitudinal Decline in Visual Memory: A Possible Protective Effect?" *Neurology* 49(1997): 1491–97.

Robbins, L. "Precipitating Factors in Migraine: A Retrospective Review of 494 Patients." *Headache* 4(1994): 214–16.

Rooke, E. D. "Benign Exertional Headache." *Medical. Clin. North America* 53(1968): 801–8.

Rose, F. Clifford, M.D. "Food and Headache." *Headache Quarterly, Current Treatment and Research* 8(1997): 319–29.

Sands, G. H., L. Newman, R. Lipton. "Cough, Exertional, and Other Miscellaneous Headaches." *Med. Clin. North America* 75(1991): 733–43.

Sarchielli, P., M. Tognoloni, S. Russo, M. R. Vulcano, M. Feleppa, M. Mal, M. Sartori, V. Gallai. "Variations in the Platelet Arginine/Nitric Oxide Pathway During the Ovarian Cycle in Females Affected by Menstrual Migraine." *Cephalalgia* 16, no. 7(1996): 468–75.

Sargent, J., P. Solbach, H. Damasio, et al. "A Comparison of Naproxen Sodium to Propanolol Hydrochloride and a Placebo Control for the Prophylaxis of Migraine Headache." *Headache* 25(1985): 320–24.

Scharff, L., D. A. Marcus, D. C. Turk. "Maintenance of Effects in the Nonmedical Treatment of Headaches During Pregnancy." *Headache* 36, no. 5(1996): 285–90.

Schoenen, J., J. Jacquy, M. Lenaerts. "Effectiveness of High-Dose Riboflavin in Migraine Prophylaxis: A Randomized Controlled Trial." *Neurology* 50(1998): 466–70.

Schwartz, Brian S., et al. "Epidemiology of Tension-Type Headache." *JAMA* 279(February 4, 1998): 381–83.

Scott, A. K. "Dihydroergotamine: a Review of Its Use in the Treatment of Migraine and Other Headaches." *Clin. Neuropharmecol.* 15(1992): 289–96.

Silberstein, S. D. "Comprehensive Management of Headache and Depression." *Cephalalgia* 18, supp. 21(February 1998): 50–55.

Silberstein, S. D. "Status Migrainosus." In: S. Gilman, G. W. Goldstein, S. G. Waxman, eds. *Neurobase* (La Jolla, CA: Arbor, 1995).

Silberstein, S. D. "The Rise and Fall of Estrogen Levels." *Cephalalgia* 17(1997): 720.

Silberstein, S. D., R. B. Lipton. "Headache Epidemiology: Emphasis on Migraine." *Neurologic Clinics* 14, no. 2(1996): 421–34.

Silberstein, S. D., R. B. Lipton, P. J. Goadsby. *Headache in Clinical Practice* (Oxford: Isis Medical Media, 1998), 1–7.

Silberstein, Stephen D., M.D. "Migraine Symptoms: Results of a Survey of Self-Reported Migraineurs." *Headache* 35 (July–August 1995): 387–96.

Silbert, P. L., R. H. Edis, E. G. Stewart-Wynne, S. S. Gubbay. "Benign Vascular Sexual Headache and Exertional Headache: Interrelationships and Long Term Prognosis." *J. Neurol. Neurosurg. Psychiatry* 54(1991): 417–21.

"Two Views on Acupuncture: NIH and SRAM Dispute Validity, Efficacy." *Skeptical Inquirer.* 22, no. 2(March–April 1998): 5–7.

Smith, Robert, M.D. "Impact of Migraine on the Family." *Headache* 38(June 1998): 423–26.

Solbach, M. P., and R. S. Waymer. "Treatment of Menstruation-Associated Migraine Headache with Subcutaneous Sumatriptan." *Obstet. Gynecol.* 82, no. 5(1993): 769–72.

Solomon, Glen D., M.D. "Circadian Rhythms and Migraine." *Cleveland Clinic Journal of Medicine* 59(May–June 1992): 326–29.

Solomon, Glen D., M.D., FACP, et al. "Hypersensitivity to Substance P in the Etiology of Postlumbar Puncture Headache." *Headache* 35(January 1995): 25–28.

Solomon, G. D., and A. F. B. Scott. "Verapamil and Propanolol in Migraine Prophylaxis: A Double-Blind Crossover Study." *Headache* 26(1986): 325.

Solomon, G. D., J. G. Steel, L. J. Spaccavento. "Verapamil Prophylaxis of Migraine: A Double Blind Placebo-Controlled Trial." *JAMA* 250(1983): 2500–02.

Somerville, B. W. "The Role of Estradiol Withdrawal in the Etiology of Menstrual Migraine." *Neurology* 22(1972): 355–65.

Spierings, Egilius L. H., M.D., et al. "Psychophysical Precedents of Migraine in Relation to the Time of Onset of the Headache: The Migraine Time Line." *Headache* 37(April 1997): 217–20.

Spierings, Egilius L. H., M.D., Ph.D., and Marie-Jose van Hoof, M.D. "Fatigue and Sleep in Chronic Headache Sufferers: An Age- and Sex-Controlled Questionnaire Study," *Headache* 37 (October 1997): 549–52.

Spierings, Egilius L. H., M. Sorbi, B. R. Haimowitz, B. Tellegen "Changes in Daily Hassles, Mood, and Sleep in the 2 Days Before a Migraine Headache." *The Clin. J. Pain.* 12, no. 1(March 1996) : 38–42.

Stang, P., and J. T. Osterhaus. "Impact of Migraine in the United

States: Data from the National Health Interview Survey." *Headache* 33, no. 1(1993): 29–35.

Stang, P., B. Sternfeld, S. Sidney. "Migraine Headache in a Prepaid Health Plan: Ascertainment, Demographics, Physiological, and Behavioral Factors." *Headache* 36, no. 2(1996): 69–76.

Stang, Paul E., Ph.D., and Jane T. Osterhaus, Ph.D. "Impact of Migraine in the United States: Data from the National Health Interview Survey." *Headache* 33(January 1993): 29–35.

Stein, G. S. "Headaches in the First Postpartum Week and Their Relationship to Migraine." *Headache* 21(1981): 201–5.

Steiner, T. J., on behalf of the Eletriptan Steering Committee. "Efficacy, Safety, and Tolerability of Oral Eletriptan (40mg and 80mg) in the Acute Treatment of Migraine: Results of a Phase III Study." *Cephalalgia* 18(1998): 385.

Stewart, Walter F. "Familial Risk of Migraine: A Population-Based Study." *Annals of Neurology* V 47(1997): 166–72.

Stewart, Walter, Ph.D., MPH, et al. "Comorbidity of Migraine and Panic Disorder." *Neurology* 44, supp. Y(1994): S23–S27.

Stewart, W. F., R. B. Lipton, D. D. Celentano, M. L. Reed. "Prevalence of Migraine Headache in the United States: Relation to Age, Income, Race, and Other Sociodemographic Factors." *JAMA* 267, no. 1(1992): 64–69.

Stewart, W. F., R. B. Lipton, J. Liberman. "Variation in Migraine Prevalence By Race." *Neurology* 47, no. 1(1996): 52–59.

Stewart, W. F., R. B. Lipton, D. Simon. "Work-Related Disability: Results from the American Migraine Study." *Cephalalgia* 16, no. 4(1996): 231–38.

Stryker, J. "Use of Hormones in Women Over 40." *Clinics in Obstetrics and Gynecology* 20, no. 1(1977): 155–64.

Teall, Judith, RGN, et al. "Rizatriptan (MAXALT) for the Acute Treatment of Migraine and Migraine Recurrence." *Headache* 38(1998): 281–87.

The International 311C90 Long-term Study Group. "The Long-Term Tolerability and Efficacy of Oral Zolmitriptan (Zomig, 311C90) In the Acute Treatment of Migraine: An International Study." *Headache* 38(1998): 173–83.

"Somesthetic Aura: The Experience of Alice in Wonderland." *The Lancet*. 251(June 27, 1998): 1934.

The Writing Group for the PEPI Trial. "Effects of Estrogen or Estrogen/Progestin Regimens on Heart Disease Risk Factors in Postmenopausal Women." *JAMA* 273(1995): 199–208.

Thomsen, Lars Lykke, and Jes Olesen. "Nitric Oxide Theory of Migraine." *Clinical Neuroscience* 5(1998): 28–33.

Thorley, V. "Lactational Headache: A Lactation Consultant's Diary," *Journal Hum. Lact.* 13(1997): 51–53.

Tokola, R. A., P. Kangasneimi, P. J. Neuvonen, O. Tokola. "Tolfenamic Acid, Metoclopramide, Caffeine and Their Combinations in the Treatment of Migraine Attacks." *Cephalalgia* 4(1984): 253–63.

Ulett, G. "Scientific Acupuncture: Peripheral Electrical Stimulation for the Relief of Pain." Part I Basics, Part II: Clinical Aspects. *Pain Manage.* 2(1989): 128–34, 185–89.

Vazquez-Barquero, A., F. J. Ibanez, S. Herrara, et al. "Isolated Headache as the Presenting Clinical Manifestation of Intracranial Tumor: A Prospective Study." *Cephalalgia* 14(1994): 270–72.

Verri, A. P., et al., "Psychiatric Comorbidity in Chronic Daily Headache," *Cephalalgia* 18, supp. 21(1998): 45–49.

Walach, H., Haeusler, et al. "Classical Homeopathic Treatment of Chronic Headaches." *Cephalalgia* 17(1997): 119–26.

Walsh, B. W., L. H. Kuller, R. A. Wild, S. Paul, M. Farmer, J. B. Lawrence, A. S. Shah, P. W. Anderson. "Effects of Raloxifene on Serum Lipids and Coagulation Factors in Healthy Postmenopausal Women." *JAMA* 279, no. 18(1998):1445–51.

Welch, K. M. A., G. L. Barkley, N. Tepley, N. M. Ramadan, "Central Neurogenic Mechanisms of Migraine." *Neurology* 43, supp. 3(1993): S21–25.

Wilson, J. R., B. H. Foresman, R. G. Gamber, T. Wright. "Hyperbaric Oxygen in the Treatment of Migraine with Aura." *Headache* 38(1998): 112–15.

Yaffe, K., G. Sawaya, I. Lieberberg, D. Grady. "Estrogen Therapy in Postmenopausal Women: Effects on Cognitive Function and Dementia." *JAMA* 279(1998): 688–95.

Index

narcotic analgesics, 21, 114, 135–37
National Headache Foundation, 32, 61, 75
National Institute of Health, 157
natural remedies, 165–72
    combinations used in, 166–67
    safety of, 168
    tips for trying, 165
nausea, 12
neck, 43, 154
nefazadone, 111, 146
neurological examination, 42–43
neurologist, 32. *See also* doctor
Neurontin, 111, 148–49
neurotransmitters, 14–15
nicardipine, 144
nicotine, 23, 79
nifedipine, 111, 144
nitrates and nitrites, 82
nitroglycerin, 23
Nolvadex, 97–98
nonmedication therapy. *See* alternative remedies
nonsteroidal anti-inflammatory medications (NSAIDs), 114, 137–38, 147–48
noradrenaline, 145
norethindrone acetate, 120
Norpramin, 115
nortriptyline, 111, 115, 145, 146
note-taking, 33
numbness, 45
nurses, 61
nuts, 80

Occupational Health and Safety Administration (OSHA), 77
odor sensitivity, 13, 68, 78
olives, 81
onions, 81
online services, 184
opiate medications, 93
Opinion Research Corporation, 174, 182
oral contraceptives, 16–17, 40, 88, 96, 99–100
Orudis KT, 94, 109, 112, 137, 148
osteopathic manipulation, 155

over-the-counter (OTC) medications, 40, 44, 132, 137. *See also* medication
oxycodone, 135
oxygen levels, 22
oxytocin, 116

pain. *See* head pain
pain relief. *See* alternative remedies; medication
Pamelor, 111, 115, 145, 146
papaya, 81
paralysis, 45
paresthesia, 9
Parlodel, 96
paroxetine, 111, 115, 146
patches, estrogen, 121, 122
Paxil, 111, 115, 146
peanuts, 80–81
Pedialyte, 12
pentazocine, 135
perfumes, 78
Periactin, 110, 115, 148
perimenopause, 118–19
period. *See* menstruation
personality abnormalities, 29
pesticides, 23, 77
pharmacist, 149
phenobarbital, 110
phenytoin, 149
phonophobia, 12–13
photophobia, 12–13
physical examination, 42–48
physical therapy, 105, 153–54
physician. *See* doctor
phytoestrogens, 120
pickled foods, 81
Pill, the (birth control), 16–17, 40, 88, 96, 99–100
pineapple, 81
plant estrogens, 120
PMS, 27–28, 89
Ponstel, 115, 148
postpartum migraine, 113–14
prednisone, 109, 114
pregnancy, 101–16
    complications of, 112–13
    concerns during, 101
    decision to have a baby, 102–3

About the Author

Christina Peterson, M.D., was initially educated as an R.N., and worked for seven years as a critical care nurse in Southern California while completing pre-medical studies at UCLA and California State University at Long Beach. She attended medical school at the University of Southern California, graduating in 1982, and completed a general medicine internship at the Huntington Memorial Hospital in Pasadena, CA. She received her neurology training at the Oregon Health Sciences University in Portland, Oregon.

Dr. Peterson has been in the private practice of neurology for thirteen years in the Portland, OR, area, and is presently medical director of The Oregon Headache Clinic in Oregon City, OR, providing diagnostic expertise and partnering with patients to explore traditional and alternative solutions to their headaches in a pateint-centered setting. Dr. Peterson is active in the local county and state medical societies, serving on the board of trustees of both. She is also a member of the National Headache Foundation, The American Association for the Study of Headache, and the International Headache Society. She speaks frequently on the subject of migraine and other headaches.